Praise for *The Accidental Truth*

"Facing the truth can be painful—but Lauri Taylor's story proves that not knowing is often worse. This is a moving, deeply felt tale."

—Dr. Daniel Amen
New York Times best-selling author of
Change Your Brain, Change Your Life and *The Daniel Plan*

"Lauri Taylor's dogged pursuit of what caused her mother's mysterious death in Mexico's hinterland has produced a remarkable manuscript about her long search for the truth despite encountering a maze of roadblocks on both sides of the American border. Taylor displays the skills of the best investigative reporters as she painstakingly searches for answers in dealing with the numerous frustrations that cops typically encounter in a cold case investigation, particularly one on foreign soil.

The Accidental Truth: What My Mother's Murder Investigation Taught Me About Life, displays all the raw emotion that besets a family when a loved one is lost to violence. It is a well-articulated and told, well-written story the reader won't soon forget."

—Pete Noyes
Investigative Journalist, Peabody Award winner,
12-time Emmy winner, and author of the
New York Times Best-Selling Legacy of Doubt,
Did the Mafia Kill JFK, and *The Real LA Confidential.*

"A captivating and compelling story of perseverance, redemption and the undying love between daughter and mother."

—Amy Bourret
Author of *Mothers and Other Liars*

"Many people fantasize about catching a thief, trapping a murderer in a web of lies, or solving a big criminal case. The fact of the matter is that most people don't have the patience, skills, or temperament to even begin to attempt such a massive task, and the professionals usually don't have the desire, time, or clearance to allow a private citizen into an investigation in any real way. However, the murder case of Lauri Taylor's mother was one of the very few exceptions to the rule. Lauri's story of how we worked together to solve this murder case is riveting and real. I dare you to stop turning the pages!"

—Candice DeLong
Author of *Special Agent:*
My Life on the Front Lines as a Woman in the FBI

THE ACCIDENTAL TRUTH

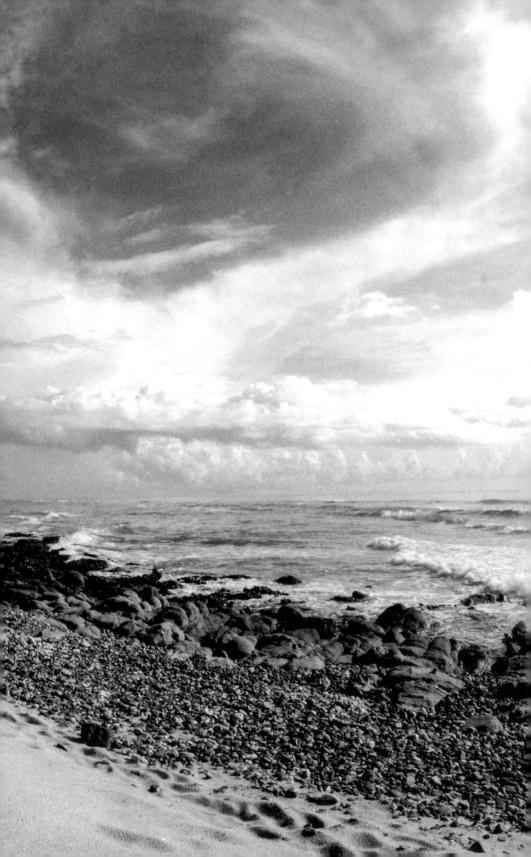

THE ACCIDENTAL TRUTH

⊱⊰⊱

What My Mother's Murder Investigation Taught Me About Life

A MEMOIR BY

LAURI TAYLOR

SelectBooks, Inc.
New York

This is a true story. All the characters and situations in it are real. I chose to change some names and identifying details of private citizens and people in law enforcement in order to protect their identity. All dialogue has been recreated from transcripts, emails or notes, or is my best recollection of events that occurred.

This edition published by SelectBooks, Inc.
For information address SelectBooks, Inc., New York, New York.
First Edition

ISBN 978-1-59079-269-8

Library of Congress Cataloging-in-Publication Data

Taylor, Lauri.
  The accidental truth : what my mother's murder investigation taught me about life : a memoir / by Lauri Taylor. – First edition.
    pages cm
  Summary: "An Orange County housewife tells the story of her four-year investigation to solve the case of her mother's violent death in Mexico that law enforcement officials declared unsolvable. Her discovery of the truth, with the help of a famous female FBI profiler, forces her to redefine her relationship with her mother and her own sense of self"– Provided by publisher.
  ISBN 978-1-59079-269-8 (paperback : alkaline paper)
  1. Murder–Investigation–Mexico. 2. Mothers–Crimes against–
Mexico. 3. Cold cases (Criminal investigation)–Mexico. 4. Taylor, Lauri–Travel–Mexico. 5. Mothers and daughters–United States.
6. Self-actualization (Psychology) 7. Taylor, Lauri–Friends and associates. 8. DeLong, Candice. 9. Criminal profilers–United States.
10. United States. Federal Bureau of Investigation–Officials and employees.
  I. Title.
HV6535.M4T39 2015
  364.152'3092--dc23
  [B]
                          2014040852

Frontispiece: desertic beach in Baja, California: image source
iStock photo © Hoatzinexp

Manufactured in the United States of America
10 9 8 7 6 5 4 3 2 1

For Clark and Katy
You are My Inspiration and My Love for You is Eternal

Contents

༄༅

Foreword

When I was first contacted by Lauri Taylor about investigating her mother's unsolved murder, I remember being skeptical (an occupational hazard in law enforcement). FBI profilers have a well-developed sense of skepticism about the tales we are told and those who tell them. We question everything and everyone. It is, after all, part of how we go about solving mysteries.

My first impression was that Lauri was in way over her head. A murder in Mexico meant that she was dealing with not one government crime-solving agency, but *two*. Lauri was not in any way qualified to do this work. She told me she had been in sports marketing, and that she was now an Orange County housewife— occupations in which people do not generally develop the skills needed to solve an international criminal case. But then I remembered, *"Well, I used to be a nurse, for Pete's sake,"* and Lauri is nothing if not persuasive.

Laypeople fantasize about catching a thief or trapping a murderer in a web of lies. From books like *Sherlock Holmes*, board games like "Clue," and TV shows like CSI, it's easy to think of crime solving like a puzzle or a game of wits. But real-life crime solving isn't like that at all. It takes interminable patience, impeccable organization, a sharp memory, a relentless desire to find the truth, and an unwillingness to take no for an answer. Most people simply don't have these skills, and besides, most criminal investigators don't have the desire, time, or clearance to allow a private citizen into an investigation in any real way. Doing so could slow down the process, lead them astray, or put them in danger—either actual physical danger or legal danger.

Lauri Taylor is *the* only exception to this rule that I ever encountered. She slowly proved to me and my fellow law-enforcement professionals in San Diego, California, and Mexico exactly how serious she was, exactly how respectful of the law and the investigative process she was, and exactly how determined she was to solve her mother's murder. Lauri swayed me, and in the end, I agreed to work with her. Being a retired FBI agent allowed me to make my own rules, and **this** case seemed worthy.

Somewhere in the midst of the investigation, I remember telling Lauri that she would have made a great FBI agent—she definitely has the chops. In the end we were lucky enough to solve the murder, but it came with a disturbing and painful price. Solving the mystery of a loved one's murder can be a mixed blessing. The truth may not be what you hoped to find, or what you imagined it might be.

During our years of working together, Lauri and I also became friends. But when she told me that she was writing this story, I was—again—skeptical. I thought that she might write something akin to a personal journal, a private account of what transpired, a few key memories. I eventually forgot about her plan until she came to me with a finished manuscript and asked me to give it a read.

Lauri's tale is masterfully written, a Rembrandt among memoirs. *The Accidental Truth* is the story of a woman's devotion to solve her mother's murder, despite overwhelming odds and international obstacles, and then dealing with the awful truth. It is woven together like a spellbinding crime thriller or a *keep-you-up past-midnight* novel. When I turned the final page, I cried, not only for the story itself, but in honor of Lauri having told it so well. I'd be lying if I let you think that this book is just another true crime story, because it's so much more than that. *The Accidental Truth* is a gripping account of a mother's sudden and violent death, her family's journey toward a painful discovery, and a devoted daughter's deliverance. It is a riveting tale—and I dare you to stop turning the pages.

—Candice DeLong
FBI profiler, author of *Secret Agent:*
My Life on the Front Lines as a Woman in the FBI,
and host of Investigation Discovery Channel's
Deadly Women and *Facing Evil with Candice DeLong*

Acknowledgments

Before I began writing this book I believed that writing was a solitary endeavor. Much to my relief, I discovered that it is a wonderful collaborative process, and I have many I wish to thank for working with me, encouraging me, and believing in me and my story.

Special thanks to my literary agent, Bill Gladstone of Waterside Productions, Inc., for taking a chance on a first-timer like me. Very sincere thanks to Kenzi Sugihara at SelectBooks for graciously sharing your years of publishing wisdom with me and for allowing my input in every aspect of my book. A warm thank you to my editor at SelectBooks, Nancy Sugihara, for your patience and thoughtfulness throughout the editing process, and for truly understanding my story.

With all my heart, thank you, Pete Noyes, for kindly treating me like a fellow investigative journalist and for graciously refusing to write this story for me. Your confidence in the merit of my story and in my ability to write it is the sole reason that I began to type the words.

Everlasting gratitude and deepest thanks to my friend and colleague, Candice DeLong. Your confidence in me throughout my mother's murder investigation changed me as a person. I am indebted to you for all that you gave me and my family—the real truth about my mother's death; although difficult, it gave us closure and pushed me to find my true purpose.

Warm and heartfelt thanks to my amazing book coach and friend, Jennie Nash. Your invaluable guidance, patience, unwavering support and stealth humor helped to transform this dreamer from a scared student into a published author, and my vague ideas into a completed book. Every word on these pages is there because you told me I was capable of writing them.

Big thanks to Dan Blank at WeGrowMedia for believing that I have something worth writing and sharing, and for helping me to authentically connect with my audience. Abiding love and thanks to Catherine

Chiesa for your treasured friendship and for believing in my story and my mental health mission with all your heart.

There would be no book without my mother, Jane A. Kling, who I love and miss to this day. She instilled in me the belief that I could be anything or do anything that I imagined. I am thankful to her for that gift and all the others she gave me in her lifetime. Among the most precious of gifts are my incredible sisters: Debbie Richardson, Sherri Holmes, and Kim Harjo who lived this story in their own heartbreaking way. I love each of you so very much and I am so very thankful to you for supporting me in telling my version of our story. What could have destroyed our family has only made us stronger and brought us closer than ever—Mom would be proud of us.

A very special thank you to my children, Clark and Katy, for understanding my need to find the truth and my desire to write this book. Despite the fact that you lived through the harrowing and unpredictable times captured in this story, you both remain compassionate, loving, and forgiving souls. I am so very proud and grateful to call you my children, and love you more than anything on this earth.

Thanks and love to my entire family for your patience and encouragement throughout the investigation and through the process of writing this book—Bob and Mary Jo Harjo, Rick Taylor, Keith Holmes, and Mike Richardson. And to the next generation of our family, may the truth help you find your way—Garrett Thurner, Adam, Tiffany and Hayden York, Mindy and Alex Goorchenko, Nick, Danny and Caroline Holmes, Amanda, Billy and Sammy Zeier, Andrew and Mia Delos, and Crystal Sorensen.

I am incredibly grateful to my fellow speaker of the truth and mental-health advocate, Sue Curran, for your love and trust in me. You will heal many with your own story, and I thank you for allowing me to share part of it here. Your friendship has helped me to close a very deep wound and to truly understand the meaning of reciprocity.

Special thanks and love to the ever-positive and always there for me, Teresa Burt and her husband Jeff. Many thanks to the dear friends who stood by me on this long journey and cheered me all the way to the finish line, especially: Carol Wilson, Jeannie Brown, Rosemary Chiaferi, Heidi

Giles, Tammy Gioiello, Lisa and Roger Sandstrom, and Kelly and Tony Wilson. To our family friends, I thank you for your generous support: Colleen Courtney Cole, Bob and Dorothy Courtney, Cynthia Beinlien-Kurt, Mel Frumes, Jodi Hempel, Brady Miller, and Megan LaRue-Kobell.

Eternal love and gratitude to my beloved friend Pam Stebbins who implored me from her hospital bed to finish this book and inspired me with her courage, strength, and love to the end. To Pam's husband, Steve, and their amazing children; Austin, Lauren, and Erik, thank you for being a constant source of joy and encouragement.

Thanks and love to the Hassett family for making me feel like one of your own: Terri, Rick, Debbie, and Katie. I am filled with pride and gratitude to Cassidy and Bennett Curran because you trusted me to tell your mother's story without fear, shame, or embarrassment. Thank you to the Schwab family for your consistent love and support.

Special thanks to the published authors who beseeched me to write and taught me a thing or two about writing: Judith Prager, Harry Youtt, and Antwone Fisher of the UCLA Writers' Program. Love and thanks to Amy Bourret who inspired me to learn and collaborate.

There were many individuals who graciously assisted my family during the investigation who may or may not have been named in this book, but to whom our family owes a world of thanks: Mike Pettit, Michael Mathe, Senator Bob Dole, The Honorable Antonio Garza, Governor John Sununu, David and Sandy Brokaw at The Brokaw Company; Jim Amormino, Orange County Sheriff's Office PIO (ret.); the San Diego Sheriff's Office, The California Department of Justice, Procuraduría General de Justicia Ensenada (PGJE), Los Angeles Police Department Cold Case Unit; Sally Cox and Adriana Uribe of Crime Stoppers, San Diego; and, finally, to the kind and caring citizens of Vista, California.

ONE

Case Closed

Many times over the last four years, I had imagined walking through the doors of the San Diego Sheriff's Office to close the case file on my mother's murder investigation. I pictured it like a movie—me, the smart, resourceful, golden child/crime solver, returning triumphantly to headquarters to hand investigators the key shred of evidence needed to convict Mom's killer. Having a vision of this ending kept me sane.

Wracked with guilt and driven by my desire to make my mother proud, one last time, I became obsessed with finding her killer, and nothing would keep me from pursuing that goal. "If you can see it, you can achieve it," Mom would often remind me as a child, encouraging me to envision being the high school homecoming queen or SMU graduate, with the promise that my unconscious brain would magically lead me to success and the coveted crown. But in this case, the answer I had so desperately searched for and so carefully envisioned about my mother's murder, and what I actually found, were two shockingly different things.

The sergeant in charge of Homicide at SDSO called to deliver the long awaited news, personally. Mom's murderer had finally been identified and apprehended, he proudly informed me, adding, that corroborating DNA evidence was indisputable, and several reliable witnesses placed the suspect in Baja at the time of Mom's death. Under the intense questioning of our devoted cold-case detective, the killer had cracked and confessed to brutally murdering my mom.

When pressed for specific details of his crime, with the hint of leniency if he told the truth, the killer coldly and casually offered that he beat Mom as she struggled to fight him off. Infuriated by the vicious things she screamed, and enraged further by the deep scratches she made on his face and neck with her long nails, he said he reached back with a tightly clenched fist, and coldcocked her above the right eye, sending her to the ground. Pouncing on her, he placed his trembling hands on her throat, and squeezed the life out of her, then left the bruised, half clothed body in the middle of a remote desert wash, and walked away.

This was the scene I had envisioned, repeatedly, for years, but it was not what actually happened. The identity of Mom's murderer was not magically served up to me and my family on a silver platter, like I had seen on CSI, where every week a murder is meticulously investigated and solved in one hour. On the contrary, we had no easy answers.

Finally, after nearly four years of searching, I walked through the doors of San Diego Sheriff's Office on January 15, 2010, holding a thin black notebook under my arm. It contained the detailed explanation of my mother's mysterious death, which I had prepared in the weeks before Christmas to present to my family and Sheriff's investigators to close Mom's case for good.

"Hello, we are here to see Sergeant Henry and Detective Nash, please," I said to the salt and pepper-haired officer behind the desk. My sister Debbie and I were familiar with the routine and handed over our driver's licenses before he could ask for them, as he always did. The desk officer smiled his thanks, signed us in, and picked up the phone to call upstairs to Homicide on the fourth floor. In minutes, Detective Tommy Nash came lumbering out of the elevator to greet us. On tiptoes, I reached up to hug him and the huge detective opened his arms wide to hug back—a gesture that always surprised me.

"Well, hello ladies, how are you? How was your Christmas?" he asked.

Debbie nodded. "We had a nice Christmas, all together at Sherri's house this year."

Over the years, I had developed good working relationships with our detectives and had learned a little about their personal lives. I felt compelled to chime in, as well.

"Christmas has to be quite a production at your house, Tommy, with six kids' gifts to buy and wrap," I said, as we stepped into the elevator together.

He laughed. "Yeah, it is, but my wife takes care of all that."

We continued to make small talk about family and the holidays as we stepped off of the elevator. Debbie and I trailed behind Tommy to the homicide division conference room, where we had had our first meeting, orchestrated by the FBI, a month after Mom's body was found. The long laminated conference table dwarfed the stark white room, and was surrounded by plush, high-backed office chairs, which under other circumstances, would have been comfortable. On the elevator ride from the lobby Tommy let Debbie and me know that we would be waiting a few minutes for Sergeant Ray Henry.

My stomach turned with the butterflies of anticipation that I felt every time I came to SDSO to discuss Mom's case. A mix of melancholy and excitement swept over me as I ran the speech I was about to deliver through my head for the fiftieth time. I had dedicated myself to this end, but the thought of giving up the hunt left me feeling oddly empty. I would be *sad* that it was over—which was sickening. After all, I had two children, a husband, and what appeared to be a rich, full life. I didn't need a murder investigation to give my life meaning, but the whole experience had caused me to feel unexpectedly empowered.

Sergeant Henry came through the door with his wide smile and crystal blue eyes sparkling, ready to be hugged, greeting Debbie first, and then he turned to me. Ray always put me at ease with his casual, sweet manner, and did not display any of the characteristics of a typical cop, looking more like a fresh-faced surfer than a seasoned homicide detective. His encouragement to our family and enthusiasm for the investigation of Mom's murder had been apparent from the second he introduced himself three years ago.

He told me to call him that day and any day I wanted to, urging me to be a squeaky wheel. He was a man of his word. I had called him many times, day and night, and he had always answered my calls. I respected him immensely for it.

Debbie and I had traveled to San Diego to thank these two kind men for their dedication and commitment to our family and for allowing me unprecedented access to my mother's murder investigation, a totally out-of-the-box approach for traditional law enforcement. They saw people like me walk through their doors every day searching for answers and closure, but what they hadn't expected was for me to treat this investigation like my business, acting professionally, creatively, and respectfully, refusing to accept anything short of total resolution, no matter how long it took.

Debbie and I were seated directly across from Ray and Tommy, a habit that began from our first meeting and continued throughout our relationship with SDSO. This set-up always gave me that unnerving "us against them" feeling, but today I felt different. I was there to share the key to the investigation and felt much more their equal than an unqualified daughter and housewife from Orange County who longed to solve her mother's murder. I had finally earned my stripes as an investigator.

I placed the notebook on the table in front of me and turned to look at Debbie, who returned my glance with a proud, knowing smile of encouragement, then opened to the first page. I breathed in deeply and exhaled with equal force, trying to push out the numbing anxiety and calm my eternally racing heart. I looked up at our two seasoned detectives and was comforted by the soft, kind expressions that I found fully focused on me.

"The reason for our visit today is to review the work that Candice has done with forensic pathologist, Dr. Michael Baden," I said, "We believe she has arrived at the only conclusion about Mom's murder that completely makes sense and is supported by the evidence we have in our possession. At Candice's suggestion, we put together an extensive report containing the new evidence from Mexico, which she presented to Dr. Baden in December. Candice and Dr. Baden, two world renowned professionals, with over sixty-plus years combined experience in their respective fields, feel, with an extremely high degree of certainty, they have uncovered the truth."

I began to review each point, just as I had explained in detail to my family only a week earlier. Ray and Tommy were silent while I spoke, but nodded their agreement at nearly every point I made. My gut told me they were also in complete agreement about our theory, which Sergeant Henry confirmed. "You hired the right person for the job," he said.

"Never in my more than twenty-five years of experience have I ever had someone from the outside come in and contribute anything to a case, let alone solve the case, which I fully believe you and Candice have done," he said.

"You should be incredibly proud of yourself," he said, and then added. "Your Mom would be proud of you."

I looked at him, half smiling, and choked back my tears. He had no idea how his words cut to my core. I could feel my heart burn, but not with the overwhelming sense of pride I had imagined and anticipated I would feel. The bitter irony was that I *had* worked all those years with the illogical hope of making my dead mother proud, but the fact was that I knew if she were here she would be furious with me, not proud. She would feel I had betrayed her secrets, and that reality left a sour taste in my mouth. All I felt at that moment was overwhelming, devastating guilt at what I had uncovered.

Squirming in my seat, I remembered that I had questions I needed to ask because our case would be closed and it might be my last opportunity to have them answered, but Debbie asked first.

"Why do you think our family was able to do this?"

Ray smiled and looked at me, "Because I found it very difficult to say no to Lauri."

We all laughed and my cheeks instantly turned a hot shade of red. Feeling my own tension ease a bit with Ray's kind praise, I asked, "Is there anything you couldn't share with us before that you can add now to support our theory?"

He turned to Tommy, who was already shaking his head no. "No, we think you have covered everything," he said.

Then I remembered one of the unanswered questions I had. "Do you have any idea about the weapon that was used?" I asked. "It is the only thing we could not find in our investigation. We understand why investigators from Mexico would not have shared such important evidence with the family, but we all wondered if you found anything unusual in the reports and photos?"

Tommy leaned in, nonchalantly clasping his hands in front of him and shaking his head. "No, nothing comes to mind, Lauri," he said, "But let me get the file and take one last look." It was so like Tommy to take the time to do something just to be kind. He pushed his chair back from the table to exit the conference room, leaving Deb and me to pass the time with Ray talking about how our family was dealing with the new information.

After about five minutes, Tommy returned, pushed the heavy wood door open, and sat down in a chair at the end of the conference table instead of taking his seat across from us. None of us expected anything earth shattering to come from a file that had been examined and re-examined countless times by law enforcement in two countries.

Deb and I continued to casually share our family's varied reactions to the revelation about Mom's death with Sergeant Henry while Tommy opened the file folder and turned the first picture over. From the corner of my eye, I saw him turn over the second photo. I figured we would sit there until he'd turned them all over, and then we would stand up and say our goodbyes—but suddenly, Tommy exclaimed, "There it is!"

I turned to see him pick up the picture and hold it up close to his face for inspection.

Ray, Debbie, and I stared at Tommy in utter disbelief. There *what* was? What could he possibly mean? Those photos must have been scoured three dozen times for evidence. Tommy launched the photo down the table towards me like a Frisbee and I felt time slow nearly to a stop. I held my breath as the white sheet turned and turned, its sharp corners cutting through the air, woosh, woosh, woosh, like the blades of a helicopter. It hung, suspended in the air for a brutally long time before it tilted up to one side then slid down perfectly in front of me.

"Oh, fuck," I screamed, "Oh fuck!" There, right before me— right where it had been all this time in plain sight—was the final piece to this dreadful puzzle.

TWO

≪δ∂δ≫

Do Your Children Know Where You Are?

Wednesday, March 15, 2006, started out just like any other day in my fairly predictable, very comfortable life as a housewife and mother in Orange County, California, but that day would be my last predictable one for many years to come. For most of the day, things were as they should be—my husband had gone to work, my kids were in middle school, and I was at home getting things done. Late in the afternoon a man came to install some shutters in the kitchen, and while I was conversing with him, the phone rang. I had no clue that the call would shatter my uncomplicated life into jagged pieces and mark the beginning of a horrible new and deeply unsettling chapter for my family and me. I just answered the phone.

"Hey, Deb, how are you?" I said, stepping away from kitchen into the living room for privacy. Because it was mid-March, I was expecting a quick chat about plans for Katy's birthday or to discuss who would host Easter lunch, but as soon as I heard her voice, I knew that this call would be different. My eldest sister sounded slightly alarmed.

"Hey, Laur," she said, "Have you talked with Mom lately?"

"No, I haven't," I sheepishly volunteered, feeling the sudden sting of guilt as I said the words, because it had actually been months since I had spoken with my mom, Jane.

"Why?" I asked, "What's up?" I was not really sure I wanted to know the answer.

"Sherri and I are going to drive down to Vista, because Laura called very concerned that Mom didn't show up for a scheduled meeting yesterday, and no one has seen or spoken with her since Monday night."

At first, I was not really worried. Debbie was simply relaying the details that she had gathered through her conversations with our sister Sherri, and Sherri's son, Adam. Mom had checked out of her life before, without much regard for our feelings, and then returned without explanation, but she hadn't done anything like that since she opened her new business. She had been very dedicated to her employees and her store, and it began to dawn on me that something could indeed be wrong. Something had concerned both of my sisters enough to compel them to drive the two hours from their homes in Los Angeles County to San Diego County to check on Mom.

"Adam went to the house to check on her this morning, and Bear and Charlie are there alone," Deb said, referring to the dogs. "Mom didn't ask anyone to take care of them."

Suddenly I knew why Debbie and Sherri were so worried. This was a red flag. Mom loved her dogs—possibly more than her children—we often joked, and quite often she brought them with her, despite the fact that Bear, a smelly, fluffy fur ball, weighed well over a hundred pounds and Charlie, the sweet lab mix, was almost as large. As far as I knew, she had never left any of her animals without care.

"She didn't ask Adam to look in on them?" I asked, certain that my nephew, Jane's partner in the A&J Consignment business, would have gladly helped out.

"No, Adam and Jane haven't spoken to each other in over a week. Mom fired Brian two weeks ago, without even consulting him, and Adam was so upset, he told Mom he did not want to be a part of the business anymore, and he quit."

Brian was my nephew's childhood friend and he had come to work with Adam and Jane several months earlier. Debbie continued to lay out the few details that she knew about the situation at Mom's home and business, and I began to realize the extent to which I had pulled back from my mother's life and how much I did not know about her work or the people that she associated with every day.

I had pulled away on purpose. The previous year around this time Mom, who had made and lost a lot of money in her lifetime, informed my sisters and me that she would like to open a consignment business. And she said that she expected us to support her in the new venture, not only by providing the start-up capital, but wanted one of us to sign the lease on a building as well because her credit was shot. The difficult truth was that Mom had walked away from basic responsibilities many times in her life—children, businesses, mortgages, husbands, and taxes. She tended to walk away when things became inconvenient.

None of us wanted to tell her we weren't willing to invest in *her*. Instead, after several phone calls between my three sisters and me, we offered to buy her a home so she could retire, live off her social security, and perhaps work as a volunteer doing something she loved. But Mom was appalled and insulted by the suggestion, and told us that she was a worker and did not want to be put out to pasture. She added that we were all too married to our real estate, having lived in our homes for long periods of time, and that she was opening her consignment business, regardless of whether we supported it or not.

The reality, though, was that she needed us, so she began to work on her girls individually, as she always did, by calling, guilt-tripping, and manipulating us until she had swayed one or two of us, which inevitably forced the others to cave in from the pressure. That is precisely what happened in March of 2005, and the doors of A&J Consignment opened with Jane's four daughters—including, me, reluctantly—as the primary investors.

My dog Bailey began to bark at the front door. "Hey Deb, I've got to run, someone's at my door. Call me back and let me know if you hear anything from Mom," I said. "Love you."

"Love you," she said, and I hung up, snapping back to my life at home. There was a UPS package left on the welcome mat, Clark had a haircut scheduled, Katy's friend Ashley was coming over to hang out, and my dad, Bob, would be arriving Thursday evening from San Francisco to spend the weekend with me. *Mom will show up, no need to panic,* I thought, and hustled to put clean sheets on the guest bed.

★   ★   ★

On Thursday, March 16, Debbie called to tell me that she and Sherri were sitting at the Vista sub-station of the San Diego Sheriff's Office waiting to file a missing person's report. My heart sank and I couldn't help but wonder if this was the right decision. *Mom will be furious with us for overreacting and embarrassing her like this when she comes back,* I thought. Debbie explained that there was still no word from Mom and that her cell phone had been found on her desk by Claire, Mom's employee at the "big store," an additional location of A&J consignment that Jane had opened back in November.

Despite the fact that Mom's scheduled days off that week were Tuesday and Wednesday, she had called on Monday to confirm plans to meet with Laura on Tuesday afternoon to write checks, but then didn't show up or call. When she did not arrive home or back to work on Thursday morning, everyone started to panic.

After hours of waiting, Debbie and Sherri finally met with San Diego Sheriff's Detective Isaac Washington and convinced him that they needed to file a missing persons report. There is no mandatory waiting period to file a MP report in California, but he explained to them that it is not a criminal act to voluntarily disappear from your own life, ignoring family and friends. Law enforcement is very limited in the action they can take when it comes to missing adults, unless there is a documented medical concern or obvious foul play. My sisters informed Detective Washington that Mom had suffered a previous heart attack and was still a heavy smoker, so she would be at risk for additional episodes. They also explained to him that she had left the home with no preparation for the dogs and with her bed unmade, both indicating to her daughters that she planned to return soon.

Mom was fastidious about the appearance of her home—always. The weekly chore list and Saturday morning cleaning ritual were rigidly adhered to when we were growing up and included very precise duties such as scrubbing tile grout with bleach and a tooth brush and raking the shag carpet, after it was vacuumed, to remove the haphazard lines in the nap created by the vacuum.

The level of Mom's obsession with the order in the home was so widely known and teased about, that my sisters' teenage boyfriends had once decided to put it to a test. They systematically turned every chair, barstool, and picture frame in our house just slightly off of square, then sat back snickering while they watched Mom return to each room and unconsciously and methodically put back every single item to its original spot. She was a stickler, with no tolerance for things out of place, and that included something as simple as making her bed every morning.

Debbie and Sherri told Detective Washington that things had been found out of place at A&J Consignment's big store, as well.

The same morning the cell phone was discovered in the store, a lamp there was also found on its side with the light bulb shattered. Not one of us girls could imagine our mother walking past a pile of broken glass and leaving it. *Was there a struggle at the store and was Mom forced to leave her cell phone behind?*

Throughout the day, I wavered between disbelief and concern that something might have actually happened to Mom. By the time Dad arrived at my house Thursday evening, I had settled on the side of concern, but a brief talk with Dad about the situation reassured me; after all he'd lived with my mom for many years, while they were married, and he knew she could be unpredictable and volatile. She had clearly just done something impetuous or spontaneous and would check in soon.

When there was still no word from Jane on Friday morning, though, Dad and I spoke with Debbie, and Sherri and decided to meet with them in Vista to develop a family plan. Packing the kids' lunches for school that morning, I noticed a shadow of concern hanging over Katy's eyes.

"Grandpa Bob and I are going to meet you at the hotel later, angel," I offered reassuringly, pulling her close to hug her. I kissed her forehead softly.

"Is Grandma going to be okay, Mommy?" she asked pointedly, pulling away to look into my eyes.

"Of course, Sweetie. Grandma probably just decided she needed to take a break. No worries, Katy girl," I said, jamming the usual turkey sandwich into her paper lunch sack, and hoping my intuitive eleven-year-old had not picked up on my increasing doubt. My instinct even then was to protect my kids from information, preserving the image of control and trying to spare them any worry.

"So I will see you tonight, right?" she said, searching my face, again.

"Right," I nodded, "just as soon as Grandpa and I can be there."

I was eager to join my sisters in Vista, so as soon as I dropped Clark and Katy at school, Dad and I got on the road to meet Debbie and Sherri at the local Denny's for breakfast.

They both seemed as relieved as I had been to see Dad and hugged him tightly as we made our way to the hostess stand. Although Dad was not Debbie or Sherri's biological father, he had helped raise them for the majority of their childhood and was the only father they knew. Over breakfast they updated Dad and me on what had happened since Mom vanished on Tuesday, and I realized that, like me, Dad needed to be brought up to speed about Mom's friends and colleagues in Vista.

Deb and Sherri shared with us that Mom's cleaning lady, Sylvia Murphy, had shown up at the house that morning nearly hysterical about Mom being gone and sobbed to them, "She was my best friend." Dad and I looked at each other completely puzzled, and I wondered if he was thinking what I was thinking—that it was strange how everyone was already convinced that something terrible had happened to Mom and odd how they all seemed to have forgotten some central truths about her character and history.

Discussing our options and logical next steps to take, we agreed it was time to hire a private investigator to guide us through this foreign process. We called my sister Kimi to make sure she was in agreement, and she offered to contact our family friend, Bob Courtney, for a referral. Bob, who everyone lovingly called, "Bubsy," was a prominent criminal defense attorney in Los Angeles and had been like a second father to Kimi and me when we were growing up with his eldest daughter, Colleen, in Manhattan Beach. Bubsy referred Chris Mendoza, a private investigator with whom he had worked on investigations out of his beachside office in the South Bay. We scheduled to meet with Chris at Mom's house on Monday.

★   ★   ★

After a long day in Vista, Dad and I returned to Orange County and pulled into the Balboa Bay Club in Newport Beach about 9:00 that evening, where my husband, Rick, was hosting his customers at the annual Toshiba Senior Classic Golf Tournament. I was thankful my kids had the comfort and distraction of the tournament, which they looked forward to attending with their friends every year, because it gave me the flexibility and peace of mind to go back and forth between Vista and home knowing they would be busy and happy.

The kids came running to greet their grandpa as soon we walked into the hotel room. It made me happy to see how much Clark and Katy loved him, especially Clark, who hugged him enthusiastically—despite the fact that he was just finishing eighth grade, a time when public displays of affection towards adults had become a bit less acceptable. Clark, a walking sports trivia encyclopedia and avid golfer, gave his attentive grandfather an astonishingly colorful and accurate review of the day's tournament standings and then quickly dispersed to the bedroom to rejoin his friends, who were playing the latest version of the Tiger Woods video game they'd brought from home.

Dad and I sat with Rick in the living area, wiped out from an emotional day, and gave him the Cliff Notes version of everything we had done and learned in Vista. I gathered from Rick's expression and tone that he was unconvinced there had been any wrongdoing. He made light of Mom's apparent disappearance, joking that he hoped she was somewhere sipping margaritas. In his defense, we had been married a long time; he knew Mom well, and given her history of checking out, had good reason to be unconvinced. But I felt protective of Mom and her memory—and afraid—and could not find any humor in the situation.

There were many things I didn't know about my mother. She was very private, but even I was surprised by the sheer volume of new information I learned about her at the house that day. One of the first things I learned was the fact that she had begun stockpiling to prepare for a possible Bird Flu pandemic. Mom was deathly afraid of contracting the bird flu and believed that the current shortage of the drug Tamiflu, an anti-viral medicine used to lessen the symptoms of influenza, could cause such chaos in the United States that citizens would panic and turn on one another like the characters from the Stephen King thriller, *The Stand*. She had amassed quite a collection of food and other provisions in the walk-in closet of her guest room.

But Mom had also taken another step to protect her safety—something totally uncharacteristic for a 68-year-old grandmother: she had purchased a handgun. In the wake of some robberies in the area, she had gone out and bought a gun, but it had not yet been found amongst her belongings. My sisters and I were also told that she had reassured her grandsons, Adam and Garrett, that when the pandemic came they should come to her house immediately and she would protect them. I awkwardly joked that I had not gotten the memo about coming to Mom's house for protection, but it was just another reminder to me of the rift that existed between us.

★   ★   ★

After a fitful night tossing and turning, I woke at the hotel early Saturday morning and I needed coffee. It had been a restless night of sleep, but I had made a decision. Although I was still both terrified and hopeful that Mom would walk through the door pissed off at how we had all overreacted, I couldn't stand by idle any longer. Throwing my clothes on in the dark, I tiptoed out of the room so I wouldn't wake my kids and their friends, who were strewn about the hotel room for a sleepover. Focused on the plan I had developed half in my sleep, I crossed the deserted lobby and grabbed a large cup of complimentary coffee from a steamy silver urn, then headed straight for the hotel business center.

In the privacy of the small bare office, I began to Google search television news stations in San Diego. This is what I knew how to do. Before I had kids, I had been a marketing professional, adept at getting media coverage for professional athletes and events, schooled in how to use a story to generate support and bring attention to a person or a cause. I could find out who to talk to and get this story on the air, and I figured that the more eyes and ears we had out there, the faster we would figure out what was going on in San Diego. Once I had developed a sufficient list of contact names and numbers, I began to make calls.

"Hello, my name is Lauri Taylor, may I speak to someone at the news desk, please?"

"How may I help you, ma'am?"

My throat tightened and I choked on the words, "My mother is missing," I squeaked nervously, sipping on my coffee to clear my throat, and swallowing my emotions as I always did.

"Just a moment," she said. "I'll put you through," and the line clicked silent.

It was the first time I had uttered those words out loud to anyone who was not in my inner circle of family and friends. Now it was real and public and quite a bit more scary. I held on the line long enough to wrestle back the tears and recover my composure, then relayed my story over and over to every newsperson who would listen. After an hour of calls, I had connected with or left messages for all the local media outlets and hoped interviews would follow. *Interviews?* I thought. *Who among us was composed enough to speak to a reporter?* And then my phone began to ring.

By Sunday word had spread like wildfire throughout the community of Vista and San Diego County that Jane had disappeared, and the ball was set in motion on a full-blown missing person's campaign. Sherri coordinated activity at the two stores, alongside Adam, who stepped back into the business to help while Sherri and I gave our first television and newspaper interviews. Talking to reporters was a harrowing and emotional task for two distraught rookie spokeswomen, but I found the media to be sympathetic and encouraging, leaving their cards and asking us to kindly update them on any news about our mother. Meanwhile, Debbie had been clever and resourceful, guessing correctly at online passwords to gather cell phone records and credit card information. Kim reached out to her network of PR professionals for advice and coordinated production and distribution of the missing persons poster, which was quickly handed out all over town.

It would not be the first time that a picture of my mom would bring me to tears, but seeing her casual smiling face sandwiched between the bold word, "MISSING" and her name, "JANE KLING," was a sit-down moment. *I really miss her,* I thought. Every step we took now felt like we were inching closer to a point of no return. The more we acknowledged her disappearance publicly, the more it became real, but I was still divided. I still had one foot planted in my life at home, where the reality of the situation in Vista had barely been acknowledged, and the other planted in Vista with my sisters who were knee deep in reality.

I went out on Sunday to the final round of the golf tournament, greeting friends, my husband's customers, and co-workers, as I engaged in relaxed conversation with kind people about the usual topics—the next dealer trip destination, someone's grandkids—and to a select few who asked why I had not attended the normal tournament activities as I had every year before,

I mentioned that my mom was missing. And I pretended that I was optimistic about her returning soon, partially because I didn't want my kids to overhear anything that might frighten them and partially because that was how I had been trained. Mom had often reminded her girls that "no one wants to hear your troubles," which was code for no matter what it looks like or sounds like in this house, we should strive to preserve our image, but most importantly preserve *her* image. This became increasingly more difficult in the coming days.

★   ★   ★

On Monday, I rolled out of my driveway, headed to meet Sherri at Mom's house. I drove on autopilot, consumed by my worry about Mom's safety and wondering where she could possibly be. I daydreamed about Mom walking through her front door as if nothing had happened. I envisioned myself running to put my arms around her, relieved that she had made it home safely. That fantasy brought a very real childhood memory rushing back into my mind.

Throughout high school, Kim and I had lived with Mom in many different areas and many different homes, and we became accustomed to picking up and moving at a moments' notice. We were thrilled when Mom picked an apartment in the heart of Manhattan Beach, one block from the sand. Mom left town quite often for her work or to visit friends (or who knows what) and Kim and I reveled in our independence. Most of the time we felt like grownups living on our own in the apartment, shopping for groceries, cooking meals, getting ourselves to school, coming and going as we pleased. This situation was ideal, until Mom would come home a week or two later and act like a real mom.

One Saturday night on a warm summer evening during one of those stretches when Mom was gone, friends picked me up at the apartment to drive me to a party. I *was* too young to be completely unsupervised at a party, but I felt like a grownup. I enjoyed my first taste of hard liquor at the home of a "boy" too old to be hosting fifteen-year-olds at a house party. As the music played, and people danced, I kept drinking, and before I knew it, I had dozed off in a chair. When I woke up hours later, my ride was gone and our host was passed out on the cool tile of the bathroom floor where he had gotten sick.

I had no cell phone; no one did back then, and it was two thirty in the morning. I did the only thing I felt I could do: I walked the four miles home, running at times because I was so afraid of being on the dark streets that late at night. Breathless from the final trudge up two flights of stairs, I put my hand on the doorknob, and panicked. It was locked. The door was *not* locked when I left and I was certain that Kimi wouldn't lock me out. *Mom's home,* I thought, and my heart began to race. Hoping that she was asleep, I foolishly tried to climb in through a small window next to the front door.

Suddenly the door burst open and Mom came rushing toward me, screaming, and grabbed me by the ponytail pulling me from the window, my hair clenched in her fist and she shoved me through the front door. "How dare you worry me like that you selfish little piece of shit," she yelled in my face, tightening her grasp on my mane. Her face red with rage, fury burning in her eyes, Mom reached back with her free hand, clutching a thin wire hanger and began to beat me.

I broke loose and ran for the stairs to my bedroom, as she yelled, "you little whore, you're nothing but a whore," her voice and words piercing me as she followed me and continued to swing. Cornered in my bedroom, I cried and pleaded, with my arms up to shield my face, and told her how sorry I was to have worried her.

Mom finally calmed down, dropped the hanger on the floor of my room, and walked out. She could hardly look at me and didn't speak to me for two weeks. The silent treatment was the punishment of shame, the message being, you are so despicable I can't look at you or speak to you. Despite the fact that she usually had no idea where I was or what I was doing, her silence convinced me that I had deserved every bit of my punishment for causing her so much agony, and I burned with shame. I never told anyone about this episode.

But now, as I pulled up the hill into the driveway of Mom's house I just wished that she would show up at the door like I had.

I forced the painful episode from my brain, wanting to think only about my good memories of Mom because I really missed her. I missed the sweet smile that lit up her face when she was happy. And I thought about Mom's own difficult childhood. She had lost her beloved coal miner father, John, to black lung disease at age seven, and my grandmother, Margaret, became a single mother. Margaret deeply favored her two sons, and sadly, she invalidated and competed with her only daughter. Jane could seemingly never do enough to win Margaret's approval, and it had caused deep resentment in their relationship.

I pushed the gearshift in park, opened my car door, and Charlie and Bear came trotting out to greet me in the driveway. I could sense the dog's disappointment as I stepped out onto the pavement. They were looking for her, too. I reached down to give them both a quick rub on the head, muttering my reassurance that she would be back soon. Both dogs trudged closely behind, following me into Mom's house through the kitchen slider overlooking her patio and the roses she loved to tend.

While sliding the heavy glass door open, a small package of white paper napkins wrapped in cellophane that lay propped in the center of the table caught my attention. I stepped closer to read the message printed in large red orange ink: "**Do Your Children Know Where You Are?**" I quickly stepped back, stung by the message.

WTF, I thought, *is this some sort of cruel joke? Or something more sinister and meaningful?* Just then Sherri walked in from down the hall and explained that she had found the peculiar napkins in Mom's buffet. My sisters had spent the last few days searching the house for clues. Mom was very private and selective about whom she wanted to know what, and it felt strange to me to be rummaging through her personal things. But I respected my sisters for taking charge of the situation and found an odd comfort in knowing that we would share the burden of Mom's wrath when she returned from wherever she was, and I would not have to face her alone.

THREE

❧

Missing Mom

Monday marked the beginning of a whirlwind week of activity at Mom's house. Chris Mendoza, the private investigator, a tall and fit ex-Marine, met us there to speak with all the sisters and officially begin his investigation. His presence in Vista was calming and reassuring to our family because of his connection with Bob Courtney, but it also marked a new point in the investigation for me. From that day on, everyone became a suspect and everything a clue. I began to look at everyone and everything differently—and it was all highly suspicious.

Chris went to Mom's stores to interview her co-workers about the details of her last day at work. Tony Coles, a compact man who often wore plaid button-up shirts, nervously relayed the details of Monday, March 13, to the PI. He told Chris that Jane had not been feeling well that morning and had a bit of a cough. She went to the liquor store just outside the back door of the big store's downtown location for cigarettes and grabbed $20 from the ATM machine to make her purchase. She left work early that day, presumably because she didn't feel well, and told him she was going to stop at the local Italian restaurant, Ciao, to pick up her favorite dish, chicken marsala, on the drive home in her new green minivan.

Tony made a point of mentioning the van, because he was part of the reason she had it. Mom's old white mercury Sable station wagon had become unreliable, so Sheri had asked if I would be willing to pitch in to buy Mom a new car for Christmas. I told her I would, and Tony helped Mom get the van in January. We paid in cash, but the paperwork for the title and transfer of the used vehicle had not come back yet. The old Sable had been missing from the store parking lot for as long as Mom had been missing, and then suddenly appeared on Sunday at the store.

Tony explained to Chris that he had lent it to a friend who saw the television coverage of Mom's disappearance on local TV and became worried that he would be in some sort of trouble for driving her car, so he brought it back to the store and parked it. Tony had nearly wept when being questioned by Chris and was later seen being consoled by Mom's cleaning lady, Sylvia Murphy, in his office. I thought their behavior was odd, but by then I had begun to think that everyone's behavior was odd.

Tuesday, March 21, Mom's case was officially moved from missing persons to the homicide division, transferring the investigative responsibilities from the small satellite office in Vista to San Diego Sheriff's Office headquarters in Kearny Mesa. The lead detective assigned to the case, Burt Long, called to inform Debbie of the change in status, adding that because we had garnered extensive media coverage over the weekend, Mom's case was considered "high profile" and consequently moved to Homicide two days earlier than the standard seven-day waiting period. I was proud of the work that my sisters and I had done to bring attention to Mom's disappearance, but the fact that the case was moved to Homicide made the whole situation somewhat scarier. Burt requested that all of the sisters meet at the house for questioning that afternoon and when I walked in the door, the house was bustling with activity.

Investigators had already been by that morning to search Mom's home and collect evidence. They had taken several items with them for analysis, including a toothbrush. I knew what they needed that for; I was completely and totally fascinated by investigative procedure and had watched enough of the OJ Simpson trial proceedings to know how important DNA evidence was to a murder trial.

They needed to gather an item to test for DNA, and a toothbrush would be more useful for this purpose than a hairbrush because saliva, blood, or flesh harvested from Mom's Oral B in the lab would give a better DNA sample than the DNA extracted from a strand of hair left on her hairbrush.

Although pleased that law enforcement appeared to be taking Mom's case seriously, and proud that I understood some of what they were doing, it was sobering to think about why they would possibly need her DNA. I didn't want my mind to go there, but I couldn't stop it. My first thought was that DNA would be necessary if they found her body and it was unrecognizable because of decomposition or, God forbid, it had been mutilated.

I sat down on Mom's couch for a moment, stunned by my own thoughts. Murder or a corpse or anything of the sort seemed completely surreal to me, and I felt like I was having a true out-of-body experience—maybe I had accidentally stepped into someone else's life because this one felt nothing like mine.

Sherri walked into the room and I stood to hug her because I could *see* how she felt.

"How ya doin, Bear?" I asked, embracing her, but she looked absolutely drained. I don't think she had been home the entire week and, like all my sisters, she was terribly concerned about Mom's whereabouts. But Sherri carried the additional weight of worry and concern for her son, Adam, who lived in Vista with his young wife, Tiffany, and their baby, Hayden. Because Adam had been Jane's partner in the business, and her disappearance occurred just a week after he quit and within two weeks of the blow-out firing of his friend Brian, Adam immediately became the focus of questions from family, the media, and law enforcement. I couldn't bring myself to ask Sherri anything about Adam or the work situation. I knew they were both getting it from all sides, so I asked about how the search by detectives had gone that morning, instead.

"They found a couple of unusual things," she said.

"Really? Like what?" I asked, now really curious.

"Well, they found a picture of Hayden in the guest bathroom trash," she said, pointing in the direction of the kitchen table to a picture of her grandson that appeared to have been crumpled in someone's hand then smoothed back out so it laid flat.

"Oh," I added weakly, not sure what to think of this strange fact.

And then she added, "Detectives also found a large amount of the prescription drug Soma in the bathroom cabinet and a huge container of Tums. They told us that prolonged use of the drug can cause stomach issues and was probably the reason for the antacids."

"What is Soma?" I asked.

"It's a highly addictive muscle relaxer."

I was swimming in a crazy pool of thoughts now, my mind racing off in ten directions with no one there to answer any of the rhetorical questions that kept flooding in. *My mother is a prescription drug abuser? What doctor did she get the prescription from anyway? Mom loathed all doctors with a passion. Except plastic surgeons. Did Soma use have anything to do with her emergency gall bladder removal last fall and was she truly in pain?* These were the thoughts that lingered with me as I excused myself to the guest bathroom. *Was my mom in pain?* I thought as I closed and locked the door behind me.

I took a quick survey of the bathroom and everything looked as it always did in Mom's homes: in order. There were clean matching guest towels hanging from the towel bar, fresh decorative soaps in the dish, and model home-type accessories and art adorning the long, narrow bathroom. It was tasteful décor, with everything perfectly coordinated and in its place. I had not yet personally touched any of Mom's belongings. I didn't have the guts to, but now I felt compelled to dig. I flushed the toilet and turned on the water as though I needed to wash my hands and bent down to quietly open the cabinet doors under one of the two sinks. The cabinet was a stuffed, jumbled mess of bathroom items and the Costco-size tub of antacids rested squarely in the center, where detectives had left it when they took the bottle of Soma for evidence.

I don't even know what I was looking for or hoping to find, or why I didn't want anyone to hear me searching that day. But sitting there on my knees peering into the dark cupboard, touching every bottle, I sensed that I would soon be digging below the pristine surface of Mom's public image into the messy interior of her real life to find the truth, and that scared the hell out me.

Detective Burt Long and another detective from SDSO arrived to interview us and brief us on developments in Mom's case. He showed us a picture of Mom from the ATM at the Von's in Oceanside where she made a deposit around 8:20 a.m. on her day off, March 14, just one week earlier. *Had it really only been one week?* She wore a red collared sweatshirt and matching sweat pants, and looked as though she had not showered or put on make up to run to the store. Investigators believed she was at the grocery store by herself, although there was no video footage available of her once she exited the store to the parking lot.

Detective Long explained to us that we would each be questioned individually and asked if there was a place for him to have privacy to conduct and record our interviews. We set them up in the guest bedroom and began to file in one by one. Although I always had great respect for law enforcement, when it was finally my turn to be interviewed I was really nervous. Sitting there in my mother's guest room, with one detective asking questions and the other holding the tape recorder, they began to push me a little about my relationship with my mom, her history of disappearing from time to time, and about her relationship with other members of my family. I was a rule follower and that meant I would be honest, but I instantly felt like a turncoat. With every answer I gave, I felt I was betraying her.

She was hardly a perfect mother, and we did not have a perfect mother-daughter relationship. She had disappeared at other times in my life, but I scrambled to make excuses for her and for myself, and for being absent from her life in the last three months. I felt like a horrible daughter even though I knew in my heart there was too much family history to explain to the detectives, and what would be the point anyway? I left the room drained and deeply saddened. I could not wait to get to the solace of my car to cry the whole way home, which I did every night that week, drying up the tears only when I reached the county line so that I would not scare my kids with my red, tear-stained face when I walked through the door.

★   ★   ★

The following morning, we learned from sheriff's detectives that our mother's old style blue and yellow California license plate that read, "RENES" had been flagged crossing over into Mexico at the Calexico/Mexicali border crossing, a little after noon on her day off, Tuesday, March 14. The personalized plate had belonged to the previous owner. SDSO also told us they had asked officials in Mexico to issue an APB and check all hospitals and morgues for unidentified US citizens. Detective Long showed us a photo of a female car accident victim, not our mother, who lay in a hospital bed in Baja, unable to speak and who had not yet been claimed by anyone from the United States.

We had gotten many tips and bits of advice since news of Mom's disappearance had aired on television. There were several individuals who called the sheriff's department and our help line to report seeing Mom's vehicle at various places across San Diego county, but all the leads had been found to be not credible, and were disregarded. *What if Mom had gone to Mexico on her own and somehow heard about the news reports of her disappearance. Would she come home?*

That scenario was far less devastating to mull over than the alternative theory being bantered about by law enforcement and my family—that Mom had been abducted and taken against her will across the border. A psychic had even called the help line and outlined a premonition. The psychic caller said she experienced strong feelings that two men had been watching and following Mom for some time and had abducted her and taken her to the Otay-Mesa area of San Diego county, a border crossing town to Mexico.

All the information that poured in was difficult to evaluate, comprehend, and disseminate to the family, and we established a pattern of sharing it among the sisters first. Whatever we wanted to share with our own families was up to us, but as the days wore on, I found myself emotionally drained and shut down by the time I arrived home at night, unable to do anything more than grunt out a few details here and there.

Pulling down the dimly lit driveway from Mom's house past her landlord Gene's home on Thursday night, March 23, I wanted desperately to escape back to my simple life: taking my kids to school and planning their birthdays, but my world was getting more confusing by the hour. I already felt completely overwhelmed when it hit me that I didn't have a card or anything special to make Katy for her birthday breakfast, which was *tomorrow morning.* Just a year ago, Mom had forgotten Katy's birthday altogether, and what made it more upsetting to me was the fact that it came just two weeks after I had sent my portion of the investment money for Jane to open A & J Consignment. Mom had plenty of time to call me back then to make sure the money was coming, but was so preoccupied with opening the store, she let her only granddaughter's eleventh birthday go by without even a call.

Wailing now, I brushed the tears from my eyes, looked at my watch, and felt slightly relieved that I would have enough time to make it to the grocery store to buy a card and cinnamon rolls before they closed at midnight. Sad and strange things always occurred with Mom around Katy's birthday, and in the silence of my car, as I focused on the long dark expanse of freeway that stretched out in front of me, I wondered if it wasn't partially intentional.

FOUR

Happy Birthday

On Friday, March 24, Katy awoke to the smell of cinnamon rolls for breakfast, with cards and balloons waiting for her downstairs. I'd managed that small gesture, but it was all I could muster the energy to do. Grandma Jane had been missing for ten days, and everything was a blur to me, the distraction so severe that I had to relinquish the reigns of birthday party planning over to Rick. Parties were my job, and I was ashamed I could not focus on my sweet girl's big day. Try as I might to protect and separate my fairytale life in Orange County from the scary truth of Mom's disappearance from Vista, I could no longer leave my thoughts and tears at the county line. On Katy's birthday, my two worlds began to collide.

I looked forward to my daughter's birthdays as much as I had looked forward to her birth. I loved planning and executing the perfect birthday for my kids. Like so many parents of our generation, I wanted to give Clark and Katy what I did not have—not just an overabundance of love and security, but fun and frivolity, as well. I wanted life to surprise my kids in good ways as often as possible, even if I had to manufacture the surprises for them. I was fortunate, because I had the luxury of time and resources to pull these things off. In his position as President and CEO of a division of Toshiba, Rick traveled hundreds of thousands of air miles

a year and booked large corporate events at hotels. He racked up
tons of bonus points and free nights. We fully enjoyed the perks of
his hard work, traveling often and staying in lovely hotels. So when
I told Rick I could not juggle birthday planning and the daily
back and forth between Vista and Mission Viejo, he took charge
and did what was the most logical thing in his mind: booked the
Presidential Suite at the St. Regis Hotel so Katy could have a special sleepover with her friends.

Birthdays are always themed occasions in our household.
Clark's were centered around sports, like his baseball birthday in
Arizona where he famously did his impression of Mike Fetters
when he threw out the first pitch at the Arizona Diamondbacks
game and had twenty thousand fans on their feet cheering. Katy's
birthdays varied in theme over the years and had become more
elaborately staged the older she got. There was the Western Murder
Mystery birthday where we each dressed up, played characters,
and even had a pretend dead body that Auntie Kimi and I had
stuffed and dressed to be discovered during the party. The year
before, we had a party based on Katy's favorite television show, *The
Apprentice.* Clark's friend Garrett played our Mr. Trump, and there
were Project Managers and team names, tasks, a boardroom for
the "firing" ceremony and even a large yellow New York taxicab
we had constructed for pictures. I took great pride in the fact that
no detail had been overlooked, and Katy and her friends raved
about the party.

This year, Katy's birthday party would be held on Saturday,
March 25. Grandpa Bob had gone home for the week, but returned
to town for the party. Kim, whom my kid's lovingly call "Auntie K,"
left Vista to join us for the birthday celebration, too—a tradition
she had started when my children were born. Katy had decided
on an "Amazing Race" theme, which took the kids on a scavenger

hunt-type of race from location to location. Dad, Auntie K, and I helped facilitate the party, but Rick ran the show, directing teams all over Orange County, including a final leg of the race on the Amtrak train returning the twelve kids to the San Juan Capistrano station where they would be picked up and taken to the hotel for the night.

Kim and I arrived in the suite at the St. Regis just ahead of the kids. Although I had traveled pretty extensively and was fortunate to have stayed in some incredible places, I was blown away by the grandeur of the room as I walked through it. There was a huge living area with floor-to-ceiling windows overlooking a lush links style golf course extending to the Pacific Ocean, with large comfortable sofas flanking a dining room table that could easily accommodate twelve people. A framed Picasso hung squarely above the massive stone mantel of the fireplace, which stood next to a beautifully polished black grand piano. I couldn't believe the painting was real—as everything in the past week was becoming all too real.

Sitting at the bench of the piano waiting for the kids to arrive, I became lost in thought for the millionth time that week. "*Where are you?*" I asked, wishing my mother would answer me. My heart was racing, the thump so intense I could feel it in my throat. I breathed in deeply and exhaled, trying to expel the feelings of fear and dread that had been welling up in me. I swallowed, trying to force my emotions back to wherever they bubbled up from. It was like swallowing a locomotive. I imagined Mom in the living room of her favorite house, sitting at her own piano, smiling her impish grin, and was thankful that I could still readily call her image to my brain.

Mom had to have that piano, a beautiful white baby grand. She insisted that it be bought in time for Christmas. Bob Kling,

Mom's fourth husband, a gruff, scruffy sailor type on the outside, was marshmallow in her hands, and so she got it. He obliged her as often as he could, with jewelry, custom homes, and a yacht, christened the "Lady J." None of it was ever enough, and Bob died (bankrupt) trying.

Perfectly polished and positioned in the living room she had decorated in her trademark cream-puff style, the white piano was purposefully turned so all who entered would not miss it as they passed through the entry of her home. She didn't play. I don't think anyone she knew played, and she had no intention of the showpiece ever being played. The fingerprints, alone, would have driven her crazy. There simply because it looked good; it was pretend. It was a prop, just as we all were in her life—placed there to make her look good.

Startled to attention by the sudden clap of the heavy front door, I smiled as calmly as possible at Katy and her friends spilled into the room, buzzing with excitement like a swarm of bees. A mix of her childhood friends since elementary school, and a handful of Clark's eighth grade buddies filled the room, wiped out from their "Amazing Race" activities. Ready for food and relaxation, they draped themselves over the sofas and chairs, the presents and cake appeared, and things seemed to be going without a hitch.

I was almost ready to relax. But after all the presents were opened, Rick and Dad pulled Kim and me aside into an adjoining room and sat us down for the conversation I had feared was coming all week. I could see it in their eyes, and wondered how I had missed it out in the other room, even amidst the balloons and the happy sounds of happy kids.

"Grandma Jane is gone. She died in Mexico," Rick gently told us.

Kim and I reached for each other at the same time, and broke into tears. Dad and Rick joined our small sobbing huddle, hugging and crying.

"What happened to her?" Kim pleaded, breaking away from my grasp.

Dad was heartbroken; you could see it in his face, but he choked out the words.

"I'm so sorry I couldn't tell you," he said, looking thankfully at Rick.

"Debbie called me this afternoon during the party. Your mom's body was found in Baja, but they are unsure about how she died."

I had noticed him on the phone quite a bit during the day. Dad explained that two people from our family would have to go to Mexico to identify Mom's body in the morning. We decided as a group that we would not tell Katy and Clark about Grandma Jane's death just then; Rick would explain to them later. We gathered our overnight bags and Rick walked us to the door.

"I'm so sorry," I blurted out as I hugged him goodbye, tears streaming down my face.

"For what," he asked, tilting his head.

I thought for a moment, the fog in my brain as thick as ever, but could not say the words I was thinking: *because this is my fault.*

"I'm sorry this happened," I cried, instead, knowing intuitively that the news I had just received had the potential to change all of us in more ways than I could possibly imagine.

★　　★　　★

Kim, Dad and I rode silently together in the car for a long while. Staring out the front window, I felt sick to my stomach. Sick with guilt, because I realized that Katy's birthday would now always fall on the anniversary of her grandmother's mysterious death—the grandmother I had deliberately and defiantly not named her after. There was something ominous about the timing, something that got at me at the deepest place in my core. I was the daughter who let my mother down and now she was dead. Those two realities bumped up against each other in my mind, like two tectonic plates crashing at a fault line.

How had I done it? In a million ways. But the big one was when I was pregnant for the second time. At twenty-two weeks, a little over half way through my second pregnancy, I found out I was expecting a girl. My firstborn, Clark, was an adorable, easygoing, loving boy and the thought of adding a girl to the family had me over the moon, with the exception of one small issue.

When I was pregnant with Clark, I was repeatedly reminded by my mother that her family "tradition" was to name the firstborn girl "Jane." She had relayed this news to Debbie and Sherri during their pregnancies, but they had boys, Garrett and Adam, and were therefore off the hook. The interesting thing about the "tradition" was that my mom was the first in her family to turn her back on it. She named her firstborn girl, my sister Debbie, Deborah Jane—a variation of the "tradition." But this was consistent with Mom's style of "do-as-I-say-not-as-I-do" teachings.

The volume and fervor of her message really amped up when I became pregnant a second time, probably because Mom saw this as her last hope of having a child named after her. But it wasn't going to happen. I didn't particularly like the name Jane, I didn't want to honor the "tradition" that wasn't really a tradition, and I was determined to name my daughter a beautiful name that her father and I both loved.

It was the first time in my life that I had chosen to do something completely for myself, without regard for pleasing my mother. The adult thing for me to do would have been to tell her long before Katy's birth that we had no plans to honor the "tradition," but I was afraid of her reaction and didn't want Mom's disappointment to dampen our excitement about having a girl. Consistent with my chronic desire to avoid conflict, I didn't say a word about baby names for nine months. Although Mom was truly thrilled and joyful when Katy arrived, her disappointment about Katy's name was evident, and I felt consumed with guilt on what should have been one of the happiest days of my life.

Driving down the highway, I couldn't shake the feeling that my mother's death on my daughter's birthday was my punishment for not honoring her and the "tradition," for not loving her enough, and for not being what she wanted me to be. But as soon as we reached the San Diego county line, like clockwork, my thoughts shifted back to what was happening in Vista and to the gruesome task that lay ahead: someone had to identify Mom's body.

FIVE

❧❧

Habla Español

I was anxious to get to Debbie because all the information I had heard so far had come second and third hand, and I wanted to hear directly from her precisely what she was told about Mom's death. When Dad, Kim, and I arrived at Mom's house, Debbie and Sherri were waiting for us, and the four sisters became a jumbled heap of tears and hugs. After we had cried all that we could, the questions began to fly at Debbie. Referring to notes she had made on a small steno note pad, Deb told us that she had received a call from Jorge Silva, the District Attorney from San Felipe, at about one o'clock in the afternoon, right in the middle of Katy's party.

"It wasn't someone from the United States?" Kim asked. "Someone from an embassy or consulate?"

Deb shook her head no. "And Mr. Silva spoke mostly in Spanish and broken English," she said.

"But you don't speak Spanish," Dad said, leaving the question hanging in the air: *They didn't even tell you your Mother had died in your own language?*

"What did he say?" I asked.

Mr. Silva had conveyed to Deb that on Friday, March 24, Mom's body was found about an hour South of San Felipe in the city of Puertecitos. He said she had died under unusual circumstances, possibly a car accident, and that we needed to have two

family members come to Mexico on Sunday, March 26, to posi-
tively identify her body.

We were all relieved that Mom's body had been found. The
media headlines of the past year had been filled with the gut-
wrenching images of the inconsolable family of a darling high
school senior, Natalee Holloway, who had disappeared on a high
school graduation trip to Aruba, and whose body had never been
found. The disappearance of a child is every mother's worst nightmare, and I prayed for resolution and answers for Mrs. Holloway,
counting my blessings that even though we weren't yet sure of how
Mom had died, I was certain we would get our answers once we
got to Mexico.

I don't remember exactly how or when it was decided that
Debbie and I would be the two designated family members to
identify Mom's body, but I knew I *had* to go to San Felipe for
many reasons. For starters, I was the only one in the family who
spoke Spanish with any real proficiency. Sherri spoke some, but
she was adamant about her desire not to go to Mexico. She was
completely devastated by the news of Mom's passing and could
not stand the thought of her last memory of Mom being the
image of her body lying in the morgue.

Sher Bear, as we called my second eldest sister, is a kind, generous, empathetic love of a person and had a great relationship with
Mom before she died. Because Sherri had been there for Mom,
supporting her financially and otherwise, in the A& J Consignment
businesses, she stood in good favor. Besides the fact that Sher was
opposed to going to San Felipe, she needed to stay behind to
manage the ever-increasing volume of disgruntled consigners and
worried employees, and to close Mom's stores for good.

I had not been there for Mom, financially or otherwise, as of
late and felt, *I really need to be there for her now.* Pushed by my guilt,

I insisted on going with Deb even though my own reservations and fears lingered in the back of my mind and caused a completely unnerving spider up the back of my neck feeling whenever I acknowledged them. Kim insisted on going to Mexico with Deb and me, as well, as did Debbie's husband Mike and Dad.

★   ★   ★

Kim and I slept, just as we had done many times as kids, in the same bed that night. We lay there sad and drained from the emotional roller coaster of the last eleven days and talked late into the night. We reminisced about our memory of becoming sisters essentially overnight, when Dad brought Kim and our brother Robbie to live with us because we were told their mother, Dad's first wife, was drug and alcohol addicted and unable to care for them properly.

Mom did an amazing job of acclimating us as a family. We were the Brady Bunch, dressed intentionally alike at all times, with matching ensembles in varying colors, and we felt instantly bonded, like a team. Mom set the tone early and we never called each other "step" or "half" growing up. Just thirteen months apart, Kim and I became very close, like twins, but opposites. Our family called us salt and pepper. I was blonde and shy, and Kim was brunette and all personality.

To Mom's credit, she raised Kim as her own, even after she and Dad had divorced. I was devastated by the loss of my mother for many reasons, but I was truly heartbroken for Kim, when I realized that Jane was the second mother she had lost in her lifetime.

It was still dark outside, and I nearly jumped out of my skin when the alarm rang. It had been a short night of fitful sleep for all of us, but Debbie, Kim, Dad, Deb's husband, Mike, and I piled into Debbie's small SUV for the 275 mile trip at about

5:00 a.m., hoping to pull into San Felipe well before noon. Our plan was to arrive early, get to the morgue, and return back home to the States in the early evening. The stretch of highway between Mexicali and San Felipe had become notoriously dangerous for tourists with robberies and even murders being reported more frequently; consequently, we were not eager to stay in Mexico after dark.

The two hour drive from Mom's home in Vista to the border crossing (called Calexico on the California side of the border and Mexicali on the Mexican side) winds up through the desert and mountains of the Cleveland National Forest, a scenic stretch of highway that rises slowly up to the Tecate divide then descends sharply, twisting and turning until it flattens out near the border. It is a peaceful but remote drive, a section of the landscape dotted with large wind turbines that look like oversized pinwheels. They reminded me of our fun childhood trips to Palm Springs that Mom loved; now nearly everything reminded me of my mom.

When SDSO informed our family that Mom had crossed at this particular border crossing, though, we were all surprised. There are three choices of border crossings at the California/Mexico border, and this one was the furthest and least convenient from Mom's home. Tijuana was only about a thirty minutes drive from Vista, and Mom was very familiar with that border crossing.

When I was in elementary school, Mom would pile all five of us kids into our station wagon for day trips to Tijuana. We hauled home the oddest assortment of fun goodies from our Mexican escapades—marionettes, piggy banks, sombreros, large colorful paper flowers, and, on one occasion, a really large green ceramic frog. I think my desire to speak Spanish may have been born on those trips, partly because I loved the way the spoken language sounded and partly because I felt uneasy not knowing what was being said around me. Mom had a great sense of adventure and was completely comfortable in Mexico, despite the fact she did not speak a word of the language.

On this grim road trip, I sat in the back seat behind Mike, who was driving, and rode with my head resting on the glass, watching the scenery whip by as I imagined Mom on the same road in her dark green Dodge Caravan. Her car had frequently—and wickedly—seemed to appear on the road next to me ever since Mom went missing, or maybe my brain was now hunting for green vans with the accuracy of a heat-seeking missile. My focus alternated between hyper alert and too tired to think. I went over Spanish words and phrases in my head, and moved in and out of the conversation in the car, as my family speculated on why Mom would go to San Felipe. To buy real estate? Because she had spent some of the happiest time in her life there with fourth husband, Bob? To buy or sell the drugs Tamiflu or Soma?

Mike had arranged for a couple he knew through his work to meet us at the police station in San Felipe to help translate for the family. They were native Spanish speakers. This came as a great relief to me, because I had not fully used my Spanish in years. Weekly conversations with my cleaning lady, Angelica, about her family in Tijuana hardly counted because we freely alternated between Spanish and English according to our comfort level with the vocabulary, and she was just grateful to have someone to chat with. There wasn't anything significant at stake so I felt no pressure to be precise. I knew things would be different in San Felipe.

When we arrived at the local police station, located in a government building called the Ministerio Público, Mike's friends were not there to meet us. I approached the desk, apprehensive and nervous. "Buenos Dias," I squeaked out in my most chipper voice, anticipating a friendly rejoinder from the man concentrating intently on the stack of papers he gripped in his hands. Pausing for an eternity, the gentleman slowly looked up from his work and met my gaze with penetrating, vacant, black eyes.

"Buenos Dias," he said flatly, staring back at me, as though I had just interrupted his lunch hour.

With family standing behind me awaiting a swift, smooth exchange, I stood there, handcuffed by panic. I could not breath and I could not get the multitude of questions that spun in my head in English, out of my mouth in Spanish. The words I had practiced in my brain for most of the five-hour drive were hopelessly and embarrassingly trapped.

"Habla Ingles?" I stuttered, praying for the miracle of conversation in my own language.

"No."

Breathe Laur, you've got this, I thought, sucking for air as I tried to formulate my next sentence. I quickly realized that I did not know the word for death in Spanish. I plunged ahead. "Lo siento," I said, "no hablo español perfectamente bien. Somos la familia de Jane Kling y venemos a San Felipe a ver el cuerpo de mi madre."

Oh holy shit, I just mutilated that, I thought. I had tried to explain that I was sorry that I did not speak Spanish well, that we were Jane Kling's family, and we had come to see my mother's body. A small flicker of recognition flashed in the clerk's eyes, but he remained expressionless.

"Tienen que esperar a Jorge Silva. El estara aqui pronto," he said. I caught the name of the district attorney Debbie had spoken to yesterday.

"Gracias," I replied, turning to my family to tell them that we had been instructed to wait for Jorge Silva who would be arriving soon. I could see the plethora of questions written on their faces, begging to be asked, but mercifully, they held them back until we took our seats in the small, quiet lobby. I explained that the gentleman spoke virtually no English and that communication was not going to be easy. Mike went outside to check on the whereabouts of his friends while the girls and I strategized about what we might ask next. When Mike returned with the news that it would be some time before Leo and his wife arrived, we all decided we could simply not wait for more information. We had to know what happened to Mom and we had to know now, so back to the desk I went.

"Mucho gusto, me llamo, Lauri. Como se llama?"

"Cruz," he said curtly, only offering his name back in response to my telling him I was pleased to meet him and that my name is Lauri. I charged ahead with my next question and asked him, or thought I asked him, if there was any written report about what had happened to my mother and if I could read it.

Much to my surprise, he said, "yes," then led our group to a tiny office just off the lobby and handed me some stapled papers. With my family huddled closely around me, I sat staring at the lines of text and scanned the document quickly for words or phrases that I recognized. The first word that popped into my mind when I touched the thick, legal-sized pages of the transcript was "sangre," the Spanish word for blood, and it was the one word that I searched for, over and over. *Where did that come from?* I thought, not able to recall ever learning the word I so desperately searched to find.

Racing through the lines and lines of text, trying to make sense of what I was seeing, the word "violencia" stopped me cold. *Violence? What kind of violence?* I could barely recall the Spanish names for body parts, which I had learned during first year Spanish, but discerned that Mom was laying on her back in the dirt when her body was discovered. Even though I could not tell my family exactly what had happened to Mom, it was apparent to me that she had not died in a car accident. For starters, just as there was no mention of blood, I couldn't find any mention of her vehicle anywhere in the report.

I was starting to sense the pinch of frustration from my family because they wanted answers and I could not give them much information. Fortunately, Mike's friends finally arrived. I was so grateful—but my feelings of relief were short lived.

Mike made brief introductions, and I handed Leo the report, which felt a bit awkward given the deeply personal nature of its contents, but we had all waited long enough, and reading from the same page I had so frantically tried to wring answers from moments earlier, Leo began to read.

"Your mother's body was beaten and bruised," he said gently, "and there were signs of a violent struggle . . . she had broken finger-nails. There were scratches in the sand . . ." He continued to speak, but I began to hear just bits and parts of what he was telling us as the numbing fog of shock settled over me, and tears streamed down my face. Everyone was crying and slumped, struck by the truth.

"Jane was murdered," Leo said.

There it is, I thought. Three words and my whole life had changed in a moment. I looked up and caught a glimpse of Dad's stricken face and knew instantly what he was feeling. He could not protect his daughters from this truth and it pained him deeply. All I could think about then were Clark and Katy. I could not protect them from the horrible truth about their grandmother's death, either, and the thought sickened me. I spent their entire lives trying to protect them from life's painful truths, the ones that haunted my own childhood. I had created a nearly fairy tale existence for them—vacations in Europe, birthday parties in the best hotels' presidential suites—but what made my stomach turn was the realization that I had done nothing to prepare them for something this awful and, quite possibly, had done them a disservice in hiding my true feelings and fears about what might have happened to their grandmother. I was well versed in unpredictability by the time I was their ages, having grown accustomed to crazy things happening in life, but they were not, and I was deeply concerned about how they would handle the news.

Cruz stepped back into the office and told Leo that the district attorney was held up in Mexicali, would not arrive until morning, and our family would not be allowed to go to the morgue until he spoke with us. We were not prepared to stay, because we all believed we were making a day trip to Mexico. Debbie and I quickly agreed that we would find a hotel and stay for the night so we could meet with the DA and see Mom's body in the morning. Mike would drive Dad and Kim home for the night and, they would return to pick us up Monday afternoon.

Mike and Dad were not the least bit happy about Deb and me spending the night there, but we were both determined to speak with Jorge Silva and get as much information as possible. Leo knew San Felipe well and recommended a small hotel just a few blocks walk from the Ministerio where we could stay and get some dinner. It was getting late, and everyone was worried about the drive home along that stretch of Mexican highway in the dark, so Mike, Dad, and Kim, drove Deb and me to the Hacienda Don Jesus, a few blocks from the Ministerio. After making sure there was a room available for us, they reluctantly hugged us goodbye in the parking lot.

"We'll be fine, don't worry," Deb said, reassuringly, stepping up to the window of the car.

"Drive carefully," I said. "We'll see you tomorrow."

"You two be careful and stick together," Mike said, sweetly.

"We promise," Deb said, leaning in to give Mike a quick kiss goodbye through the window.

★   ★   ★

In the lobby of the Hacienda Don Jesus, the hum of a large fish tank that framed the wall behind the reception desk was temporarily drowned out by the shriek of the large bird perched in his white wire cage in the restaurant adjacent to reception area. When signing my credit card receipt and collecting our room keys, I wondered to myself, *Did Mom stay here last week and should I ask the desk clerk if he had seen her?* But the sympathetic expression on the man's face told me that he had likely already guessed why we were there.

Our simple second floor room had two double beds with old-fashioned floral bedspreads, pushed against poured concrete headboards that were separated by a small oak nightstand. A plastic shower curtain hung from the rusted bar of the tiled shower in the small bathroom. While Deb washed her face in the small porcelain sink, I propped myself on the bed for a minute, closing my eyes and laid my head back against the cool concrete because the only chair in the room was a hard wooden model, tucked in front of a small desk by the door. A large ray of sunshine spread across the floor at the foot of my bed; it came through a two and a half-inch gap between the door and the non-existent threshold. Every footstep and every word from outside could be heard through that gap.

Debbie and I decided we better do our errands in town before it grew dark. We were both afraid of being on the streets at night, even though San Felipe was known as a perfectly safe tourist destination. Feeling completely drained, we needed caffeine and wanted to hunt down some basic toiletries since we didn't bring so much as a toothbrush with us.

Leaving the room, I pushed the button lock on the center of the door handle and lost my breath for a minute because I realized that the meager lock could be all that separated Deb and me from the person who had murdered our mother.

We wandered the quiet, seemingly peaceful, sand-covered streets for a few blocks until we found a small strip center with a liquor/convenience store next to an ice cream shop with a sign in the window that that read "Café." Deb and I shopped at the liquor store first, grabbing toothbrushes, toothpaste, deodorant, a comb and a tiny bottle of Jergen's lotion, then stepped next door to get our coffee. I was nearly overjoyed to read the menu above the freezer case listing the coffee drinks they offered, including my favorite vanilla latte. In a place where everything was scary and unfamiliar, the smell and taste of the warm rich coffee was extraordinarily comforting. Deb and I took our drinks "para llevar" (to go) and walked back to the hotel just before the sunset.

❧❧

SIX

Deep Purple

I heard the click of the skimpy lock and the turn of the door handle and sat up in the bed, rubbing my eyes. Debbie stood at the foot of the bed smiling down on me with a large steaming Styrofoam cup in her hand. After dinner in the hotel restaurant, we had laid in our own double beds chatting late into the night, crying and laughing, sharing stories about our rollercoaster of a childhood, remembering the crazy and the good, just like I had done on Saturday night with Kimi at Mom's house. Deb was the keeper of the family history, she knew all the names, places, and stories, and I found comfort in hearing them, even the ones I already knew.

"Thanks, Deb, I said, smiling and reaching for the fresh cup of coffee. "You remembered." I had half jokingly warned her during our night-time conversation to not even attempt to speak to me in the morning until I had my cup of coffee. "It would be useless," I said, because I needed the caffeine to think properly, and on a day when we had to go to the morgue to identify our mother's body, a large dose was definitely needed.

We ate a quick breakfast in the restaurant of the hotel and walked over to the Ministerio Público where we hoped to meet with the district attorney. My stomach turned from the anticipation and fear of what lay ahead. Cruz, who was no happier to see

us today than he had been the previous day, instructed us to take a
seat and wait, which we did, for forty-five long minutes.

Finally, a tall, distinguished gentleman strode through the door.
It was obvious from his gait and attire that he was someone of
authority. Nicely dressed in slacks and a collared shirt, and carrying
what appeared to be a briefcase, the gentleman simply nodded to
Cruz as he made his way to the back of the Ministerio and disappeared down a hallway. A few minutes later, Cruz came and got us
and walked us back to the office of District Attorney Jorge Silva,
the man with the briefcase. He stood as we walked into his office
and extended his hand over the simple metal desk.

"Mucho gusto, Jorge Silva," he said, shaking Debbie's hand.

"Hello, I'm Debbie."

"Much gusto, soy Lauri." I said, nervously, shaking his hand.

"Habla español?" he asked me. He seemed hopeful.

"Si, un poquito pero entiendo mas que puedo decir," I said.
I speak a little Spanish but understand more than I can say.

With the invitation, the district attorney plowed forward in
Spanish, his accent and rapid delivery making it difficult for me to
pick out and understand more than a few words at a time. I was
tempted to ask him to write down what he was saying, but politely
asked him if he could speak more slowly, instead. Concentrating on
his face so as not to miss a word, I followed his eyes, as he lowered
his head and looked down into a manila file folder that lay on the
desk in front of him. Along with the typewritten pages that he casually leafed through, I noticed several Polaroid photos stapled to the
top edge of the file. I closed my eyes, trying to un-see what I had
instantly realized were pictures of my mom, the outline of her body
unmistakable, even from across the desk. Debbie noticed the photos
at the exact same time. My chilaquiles breakfast was instantly in my
throat. I looked away to try to regain my composure and saw two

brown plastic grocery bags filled with plastic drink bottles on top of a low file cabinet. They were covered in black fingerprint dust.

Just then, Cruz popped his head in the door and the DA got up and walked out.

Deb turned to me. "Laur, we need to see those photos," she insisted.

I knew she was right and I knew it was silly for me to resist, given the fact that I was going to see Mom's body, up close, in the flesh, within the hour, but I looked at my lap and shook my head, no.

"Sweetie, we have to . . ." she prodded, gently.

I nodded. "Look at those," I said, pointing to the sacks. "They look like evidence."

"Let's ask him when he comes back."

As though he had heard us, Jorge Silva walked back in the door and we tried to resume our stilted conversation. Although he was difficult to understand, when the DA put Mom's purse on the desk, it was obvious he was going to allow us to look through it. Deb and I rummaged through it quickly and found Mom's wallet, a small blue notebook, Deb's business card that the DA had gotten her number from to call about Mom's death, and a scrap of paper on which was written both Sylvia Murphy's phone number and my phone number.

When we had finished with the purse, though, and tried to delve back into the facts, it was very apparent that our communication of this incredibly important topic was not going well and that we would need a translator. Deb and I agreed to wait until one was available and took our seats back in the lobby. Feeling the glares and the stares from the others in the room, I wondered if they all knew why we were there. A tall man with a kind round face and a head full of tight dark curls, smiled in our direction. I had noticed him earlier while we were waiting and felt his curiosity. I smiled back weakly, and he walked over to introduce himself.

"Hello, I'm Octavio. How are you?" he said, offering his hand.

Relieved to hear his perfect English, Deb and I jumped to our feet to shake his hand and poured out our sad tale. Octavio, who was the local pharmacist, listened intently and offered to translate for us. The three of us walked over to Cruz's desk and Octavio told him that he was willing to act as our translator. We were escorted back to Jorge Silva's office to continue our conversation.

The first thing Deb asked Octavio to tell the DA was that we wanted to see the photos in his file, and we wanted to know if the grocery sacks had something to do with Mom's case. A surprised look covered the DA's face as he spoke back to Octavio, telling him that the bottles had been collected from the crime scene and fingerprinted. After explaining this, he handed the file with the photos to Debbie. She leaned over to me and we glanced at the pictures together. Mom was indeed on her back, half clothed, bruised, both hands conspicuously covering her bare chest, and her bare feet exposed in the dark sand. It was awful to see Mom like that, but Deb was composed and businesslike, and inexplicably, we discussed what we saw and kept our emotions in check.

"I think those tattoos on her chest are new, Laur."

"I guess we will see for ourselves soon enough."

How the hell could this have happened? I thought to myself. Octavio continued to translate the DA's words as we carefully examined each photo. "Your mother was strangled, she put up a fight, there were scratch marks in the sand . . ." his words trailing off, but sinking in, and stinging. I pictured the scene in my head and cringed, envisioning my feisty mother, using her signature long painted nails that I had so admired as a child, to battle for her life.

"Can you ask him if they scraped her nails for DNA," I asked, struggling to exhale.

Octavio asked my question and told us that the DA would check with the medical examiner. The DA also informed us that investigators from Ensenada were spending the day in Puertecitos, which was within their jurisdiction, visiting the crime scene and interviewing locals. We were told that we would be allowed to go identify Mom's body within the next few hours, but that the Ensenada detectives had requested for us to remain in San Felipe for questioning. The "request" though, sounded more like, "you are not allowed to leave Mexico until they say you are allowed to leave Mexico." Deb and I were so distracted by the fact that we had been vaguely told we were going to the morgue soon, that the new information barely registered with us, until our ride home showed up.

Dad and Kim had driven from Vista to San Felipe for the second time in twenty-four hours, and the minute they arrived, we had to tell them all the new information we had just learned and that we would not be returning home with them, again. Deb and I weren't exactly sure when we would be leaving Mexico. The landscape at the Ministerio Público seemed to change with the wind and we had to remain flexible.

Dad and Kim had planned only for the day, based on what we had told them on Sunday evening, and did not bring anything with them to stay, including Dad's medication, which he could not go without. They reluctantly drove away from the Ministerio, but only after Deb and I reassured them we would figure out how to get home later. We marched back to our spots in the lobby to wait. For the next hour, Deb and I waited until Cruz motioned me over to his desk and told me the DA had finally given his permission for us go to the morgue.

The moment we had anticipated and dreaded for the past twenty-four hours had finally arrived, and we had no ride to the morgue. It was too far across town to walk, and the thought of hailing a cab from the police station to the morgue seemed absurd and impossible. The cabs were centered downtown, chauffeuring happy relaxed tourists from the hotels to the bars, restaurants, and beaches. There was no one waiting out front of the local police station for Debbie and me; we were all alone, isolated by miles, circumstance, and a language barrier.

Once again, and eerily as if on cue, Octavio, our pharmacist–turned-interpreter, stepped in to offer us his assistance.

"I can take you there," he said, "My car is outside."

Debbie and I exchanged worrisome glances. We had just met Octavio a little over an hour earlier. He seemed kind and genuine, but I could not shake the feeling that he had been watching us a little too closely as we sat in the lobby of the Ministerio. I felt suspicious of everyone, and it seemed as though everyone was suspicious of us, but we needed help and he was the only person there offering it. As much as we dreaded what we were about to do, Debbie and I were both eager to get it over with. We had a list of questions we hoped would be answered by seeing Mom's body, so we didn't hesitate to accept Octavio's offer.

"Thank you," Debbie said, "You sure you don't mind?"

"We'll need a ride back, too," I offered, apologetically.

"No, no problem," Octavio said, dangling the keys from his hand.

Octavio pushed open the glass door of the Minesterio Público and strode confidently through, with Debbie and me following closely behind.

Walking out into the sunshine for the first time since early that morning, I was reminded that we were in a sleepy Mexican resort town. A warm breeze washed over me and I breathed in the fresh salt air, thinking, *Mom always loved the smell of the ocean,* and swallowed the lump that grew in my throat. Just blocks from where we were, the streets and the beachfront Malecon would be filled with the tourists and "snowbirds" from the United States and Canada, who flocked there for the temperate climate and affordable beach living. The city that boasted the slogan "No Bad Days" had not yet lived up to its motto, in my estimation, as this day seemed to be moving from bad to worse by the minute.

The street and sidewalk were unusually empty, leaving me to wonder if the old "siesta" tradition was observed in San Felipe. Octavio's banter slowly began to pick up as we walked towards his car. I wasn't sure who he was trying to make more comfortable by filling the silence, but I was relieved either way because it meant I wasn't forced to make polite conversation or translate anything. Parked at the curb, Octavio's circa-1980 Trans Am was wrapped in a thick blanket of Sea of Cortez dust. A slightly gothic-looking, fire-breathing bird adorned the hood, and peeked its head through the layer of soot, covering our dark purple ride.

"This is it," he said, with a wide, proud smile, waiting for our enthusiastic reaction.

Debbie and I nodded and earnestly chirped, in unison, "It's great, thank you."

Octavio held open the passenger door and moved the seatback forward to make room for one of us to climb in.

"I'll jump in the back, Laur," Deb said, stepping into the narrow backseat, strewn with an assortment of beer cans, bottles, and food wrappers. The beige lining of the vehicle's roof, torn from its seams, hung down like a privacy curtain, separating the front seat from the back. Without a word, Deb simply whisked it out of her way, and sat down, holding it next to her ear so she could see us. I slid into the passenger seat directly in front of her while Octavio jumped behind the wheel and turned the key. The car started with a roar, and the loud noise sent my heart racing.

As we pulled away from the curb, Octavio shouted over the sound of the engine. "My wife asks me all the time, 'Tavo, when are you going to wash your car?' I give her the same answer every time, 'I'm a Mexican, we don't wash our cars!'"

I burst out laughing, thankful for the levity and the momentary distraction from thinking about where we were headed, but I was instantly struck with a feeling of regret. *This cannot possibly be the way someone should behave on the way to the morgue,* I thought, admonishing myself for the slip.

Octavio just shrugged his shoulders at his own joke, smiled his toothy grin and pulled out onto the street. The warm dry Baja air blew over us through the open T-top as we cruised through town, hair flying in every direction, the shredded fabric of the roof flapping loudly and the dust of the sandy streets billowing up behind us. It was difficult to hear Octavio as he proudly pointed out the sights of the small resort town, one by one.

Octavio explained that San Felipe had been a fishing village once, but now more of the city's revenue came from tourists and retirees. Only half listening, my mind was fixated on the task at hand. *This is completely surreal,* I thought. *I am driving to identify my mother's dead body.* I tried to be attentive and soak in the information Octavio was so proud to share as the pseudo-ambassador of San Felipe, but all I could think about was what the awful moment ahead of us might be like. I watched the run-down homes of the residential area we drove through, but what I saw was me standing over a table where Mom's body lay, and the questions began to stream out as quickly as the scenery we passed. *Will she be zipped into a black bag, like the ones I have seen on TV so many times? Will she have a toe tag with her name on it, not Jane Doe, but Jane Kling? Would*

I throw myself over her, like the grief stricken relatives I have seen do at open casket funerals, knowing it would be the last time I could touch my mother?

My eyes welled up, I fought back the tears, and my throat began to tighten. It was all I could do now to remember to swallow and breathe. Octavio was just finishing up telling Debbie and me how he had named his children after the original members of the band Deep Purple, Ian and Steve, when we pulled up to a small wooden building.

We got out of the car, climbed the creaky planked stairs at the front of the office and opened the door. Sitting at a large desk, behind what looked to be a Depression-era typewriter, was our medical examiner. He smiled weakly as we stepped up, hands outstretched to meet him.

"Buenos Dias," he said in our direction, reaching out to shake Octavio's hand first, as if they were old friends. Octavio kindly introduced us.

"This is Pablo Meza," he said.

"Mucho Gusto, Pablo," I said, shaking his hand.

He smiled broadly with sympathetic eyes, exposing his jumbled brown teeth. His smile was his acknowledgment of my effort to address him in Spanish, and put me at ease. He motioned for Debbie and me to sit in the two seats in front of the desk. As we had so many times in the past two days, Deb and I looked at each other, comforted by knowing that we knew the other was thinking the exact same thought: *How the hell did we get here to the Twilight Zone? And no one will ever believe this when we tell them.*

Pablo reached over, opened a drawer, carefully placing a pre-printed form into his typewriter. Speaking to us in English, he asked, "Mother's full name?"

"Jane Alice Kling," Debbie answered.

Pablo looked up from the typewriter, pleading with his eyes for help and Debbie began to recite the letters.

"J," click.

"A," click.

"N," click.

"E," click, until she had spelled out Mom's entire name for him.

Pablo slowly pecked out the remaining answers on Mom's Official Death Certificate with the pointer finger of his right hand, and then handed it to us for our signatures—and that was it. With the paperwork complete, there was nothing left to do but see her body.

Pablo, Debbie, and I walked out the back door through a small courtyard area to what appeared to be an attached garage, leaving Octavio behind in the office. The metal building seemed an afterthought, loosely clinging to the office building and resembling the type of sheds sold at Home Depot, with a rusty corrugated roof and windows that were opaque. Deb reached over to squeeze my hand as we walked shoulder to shoulder, ever the reassuring big sister, but then we had to separate so we could pass through the door. Pablo stood there, kindly holding the door for us.

Stepping into the coolness of the dimly lit shed, I scanned the area quickly, vowing to remember every detail of the moment so I could share it with Sherri and Kimi at home later. My first thought as I walked in was *bomb shelter*. The cool air, faint smell of earth, and sparse lighting made me feel as though we were underground. Several open coffins were scattered across the room, some propped on their sides leaning against a wall and awaiting their occupants. I shuddered.

Was this the room where they performed Mom's autopsy? It was hardly the sterile, clinical space where I had envisioned them carefully assessing her injuries and collecting valuable DNA evidence. The room seemed more suited for potting plants than for the serious forensic work that I had hoped had taken place there, but knew instantly, had not. We stopped in front of the large industrial refrigerator that hummed in the corner of the room, and suddenly I realized that this was where Mom's body was being kept. I felt lightheaded. Had I been holding my breath the entire time? I gulped down a huge breath of air through my mouth, because I was so afraid of being overcome by the smell of death, and moved closer to Debbie as Pablo reached for the large handle of the stainless steel door.

He opened the heavy door and gently pulled a large tray from the middle of the fridge. Fearful of accidentally seeing the bodies of other victims occupying the fridge, I forced myself not to look up or down from the tray in front of me, focusing intently on the thin blue sheeting that loosely covered my mom.

I could hear Debbie's voice faintly in the background explaining to Pablo that we wanted to see her whole body, not just her face. Just then, I felt as though I had fallen into a well, as Debbie's words and Pablo's responses echoed around me. I struggled to be present in the moment, concentrating on Pablo's baffled and concerned expression.

I am sure he was wondering why in the hell we would ever want to see her whole body, but assured us we could see whatever we wanted to see. His large brown hand reached down across the fabric and pulled it back, exposing Mom's bruised and swollen face. Deb snapped her eyes towards me with a pained, yet sweet expression, her mouth curling up as it always did when she was about to cry, then she quickly looked back at Mom, holding back her tears.

The deep dark purple color of the bruise that covered Mom's left eye stood out like a beacon in contrast to the thin porcelain skin on her face. Just beneath her eye, which was thankfully closed, the flesh of her bruised cheek bulged up as if it was about to burst.

I had so feared Mom's eyes would be open and my memory of her sparkling, happy, brown eyes would be forever replaced with dead, staring eyes. Her short pale-strawberry blonde hair was thin and faded. I tried desperately to remember every detail of what she looked like as I scanned her face for clues. This was it, my last chance ever to see my mother. A small scrape, about the size of a nickel, grazed the skin just below her lip. A pale blue baseball cap with a San Felipe logo on the front lay on the tray next to her head and seemed wholly out of place. *Whose hat was it? Mom wouldn't buy, let alone wear, something like that,* I thought.

The skin on her neck appeared to be heavily bruised from just below the ear around to the front of her neck, especially at the base, where her throat met the top of her chest. *Who could have done this to her?* I wondered, imagining large hands tightly wrapped around her throat. I swallowed the large lump that welled up in my own, and my eyes followed her collar bone across to another large bruise on her left shoulder, then down her arm which was laced with scrapes and scabs across much of her forearm and hand. We had been told that she had defense wounds; she had broken nails defending herself.

Debbie asked Pablo to move the drape back further so we could examine the tattoos on Mom's chest that we had seen in the crime scene Polaroids. They appeared to be new tattoos. Thin black ink outlines were covered in vibrant green leaves that had small yellow rosebuds attached, forming matching rosebush "wings" over her right breast, and covering part of a mastectomy scar of her left breast. Mom's breast had been removed when she had cancer ten years before, and I was convinced that she'd gotten the tattoos as an effort to feel beautiful. Before her diagnosis, she had been one of the first women I knew to get breast implants, and she took great pride in her appearance.

Losing one of those breasts had to have been one of the most painful, humiliating moments of her life. It made sense that she would get yellow roses tattooed there. Yellow roses were always her favorite. Seeing the image on her chest made me extraordinarily sad, not only because Mom had had to endure the indignity of breast cancer, but also because she felt the need to keep the tattoos a secret from me.

Debbie had her own thoughts about why Mom would have new tattoos, and she was convinced it was because there must be a new man we didn't know about in Mom's life. *Did she follow a man to San Felipe? Did she have the tattoos done in San Felipe?*

"Pablo, we need to see it all," Debbie said, as she directed Pablo to pull back the cover even further, exposing the lower half of her body.

As the drape flew back, Debbie and I both stared, bewildered at the line of tattoo that stretched across Mom's pelvis from hip to hip. The same thin black ink outline as the chest tattoos covered her skin in a much bigger pattern, with larger green leaves, blooming yellow roses and floating butterflies at each hip bone. Suddenly I felt embarrassed and ashamed that we had allowed Pablo to see our mother like this, as if he wasn't already intimately aware of every inch of her autopsied corpse. She had so many secrets, and I felt enormous guilt for exposing them. Mom had trained me better. All I wanted now was for this to be over. I felt incredibly relieved when Debbie told Pablo we had seen enough. I had seen enough for a lifetime.

SEVEN

What We Left Behind

Debbie and I had naively believed that our trip to the morgue would provide us with answers about Mom's death. But, in fact, the opposite occurred, and our list of questions grew, not only about her death, but about how Mom had lived her life. The tattoos had bothered Debbie because she believed that they indicated a new man in Mom's life, someone who might have been a threat to Mom, but they bothered me for an entirely different reason. Mom had hidden her tattoos from me, and from most of the world, and was the living image of a conservative grandmother, by all accounts, in speech, dress, and political affiliation.

Although I knew she had some tattoos, since I had seen them peak out of her clothing before, I was acutely aware that she did not want me to see them because I watched her nervously pull at her clothing to cover them in my presence. I honored Mom's desire to keep her tattoos private, never asking about them, but felt sad that she did not feel comfortable in her own skin with me. As we walked with Octavio from the morgue back to his car, my mouth went dry and I was soaked in a sea of dread about the work that was in front of us. We had to find a way to get Mom's body back to the United States, and something told me that I had much more to learn about my mother's life before I could uncover the truth about her death.

Debbie asked Octavio to drive us to the nearest tattoo shop. His confused expression begged to ask a question, but neither of us was in the mood to answer. We needed to know if Mom's tattoos were recently done, because she may have come to San Felipe for that reason. I dialed my friend Craig, who was a contractor working on our remodel. He was the only person I knew with extensive knowledge about tattoos, and I felt comfortable he would answer my questions without judgment.

"Oh my God," he answered, "How are you?" His concern, apparent in his tone, told me Craig had gotten the memo that Mom's body had been found.

"I'm okay, thanks. How are you?"

"I'm good. Where are you?"

"I'm still in Mexico with my sister, but I have to talk quickly because our phones are running out of battery. Can I ask you a few questions?"

"Of course."

"Debbie and I just left the morgue."

Craig let out a low groan, but I kept talking.

"My mom had a line of tattoos from hip to hip, above her pelvis. Debbie and I are trying to determine how recently she got the work done and where she got it done."

"So she had a porno-belt?"

"What did you say?" I asked, knowing the answer, but needing him to say it again for confirmation.

"A porno-belt, Laur, that is what it's called."

I gasped for breath, pressing forward through the embarrassment that all children feel when they have to acknowledge their parents are sexual beings, something that still felt odd to me, even in my forties. Fearful that my phone was about to die, I pressed on and asked Craig to tell me quickly how I could tell if Mom's tattoos were new. He asked me to describe what Mom's looked like—the skin around the design, the color, and the heaviness of the outline. He explained that tattooing is an art, and that each artist, has a distinctive style, which differentiates their work from others. He suggested that describing that style might be a way for us to find the place where Mom got her work done. I thanked Craig and scrambled off the phone to relay the information to Debbie before we walked into the tattoo shop.

In our first attempt at investigative work, Deb and I peppered the reluctant shop owner with questions, and although he was polite and sympathetic, he had very little to say to us. Who could blame him? There were client privacy issues to consider and to make matters worse, we had blurted out, far too quickly, that our mother had been murdered near Puertecitos. It was hard to say, let alone, believe, and we struggled anxiously to come to grips with all that we had learned in such a short time.

Deb and I both needed to decompress, and we needed food, so we headed towards the Malecon in the center of town on foot. We silently traversed our way through the streets of San Felipe until we found a little restaurant with an outdoor patio overlooking the Sea of Cortez. Thankful when the server greeted us at our table with a fresh basket of tortilla chips and homemade salsa, we gratefully ordered two beers, and hoped they were cold. Parched from the walk in the heat, we languished in our chairs for a bit until our drinks came, even though we had so much to talk about and so much to communicate back home to Sherri and the rest of the family.

They were working on plans for Mom's memorial, which we were holding in less than a week, and were waiting to hear from us about Mom's body. Peeling the soggy label from my bottle, I stared at the blown-out, blue waves across the street. Debbie had already jumped on the phone and was chatting with her husband when my phone rang. I glanced at it and saw the name Ben Cook flash across the screen.

Sherri and I had given our first television interview to Channel 8 when Mom was missing and Ben Cook was the cameraman on the shoot. Medium build and balding, Ben was a warm, empathetic, fatherly guy, and he put Sher and me both at ease, sensing our anxiety about being on camera to talk about Mom. He gave me his business card when the interview was over and asked me to call him if we got any new information on the case. I certainly felt like I would call Ben first if there were anything to report. I liked him. I picked up the phone.

"Hi, Lauri. How are you?" This Ben from Channel 8."

"Hi Ben, I'm okay, thanks," I fibbed.

"We have gotten word here at the station that your mom's body was found in Mexico. First, let me say how sorry I am for your loss."

"Thank you," I offered, but I was suspicious, sensing that "offering condolences" was not the reason for his call.

"We are thinking about sending a news truck there to cover the story," he said.

"No, no, Ben. There is nothing to report from here."

I could hear him pause. "Lauri, we have acquired some crime scene photos of your mother taken by an American woman living near San Felipe . . . and we are going to put them on the air tonight."

I closed my eyes and lay my head in my hand, pressing the phone to my ear, unable to breath, suffocated by what he told me. *I have just left the morgue and I am downing a barely cold Pacifico in an attempt to dilute the all-too fresh images of my mother's bruised face from my brain and he is telling me this now?* Seized by disappointment because I had foolishly trusted a member of the news media, I was determined not to offer Ben any new information. I was incensed and screamed back at him, alarming Debbie, who ended her call and stared at me in disbelief as she listened in.

"You've got to be kidding me, Ben. Why? What good could this possibly do now? I have teenaged children who can Google their grandmother's name and see whatever you broadcast."

"I'm sorry, Lauri."

"I've got to go," I said, cutting him off and thought, *I need to warn my family*.

Debbie sat nervously, her eyes pleading for an explanation. She could sense my rage.

"Mother Fucker," I bellowed at Ben, and then slapped my flip phone shut.

I shook as I repeated everything I had just been told. Debbie looked at me like I had a third head.

"I've never seen you speak to anyone like that before."

"I had to. This could hurt my kids, our family."

We sat, quietly sipping our beers for a moment, and absorbed the latest round of emotional trauma in what was starting to feel like a very lopsided prizefight. Debbie and I picked at the large plates of food that had sounded pretty good when we ordered them, but had swiftly lost their appeal.

"We better call home now, Laur," Debbie said, placing her napkin neatly on top of her barely touched plate.

"Okay," I squeaked, drained by the exchange with Ben, but thankful that my big sister was there, as she always had been for me, to direct the show and keep me focused on what we needed to accomplish—bringing Mom home.

After lunch, we walked back to the Ministerio to wait for the detectives from Ensenada to arrive, eager to speak with them because Pablo Meza from the morgue had told us that Mom's body could not be released without their permission because they had jurisdiction in the case. Debbie and I sat close to one another in the lobby while she placed the call to Sherri to warn her about the photos being aired on TV that night in the San Diego area. She was as surprised and pissed as Debbie and I had been, and was equally disappointed in Ben Cook.

"Sher," I overheard, Deb ask, "have you heard anything yet from Detective Long about having Mom's body brought to San Diego for an autopsy?" She paused to listen. "Okay," she said, "we will call you after we talk with the investigators about releasing Mom's body to us."

She hung up, but before I could ask Deb about Sherri's conversation with Detective Long, Jorge Silva came walking through the lobby, and we sat at attention in our chairs. He smiled and held up what appeared to be a Ziploc baggy next to his ear as he continued to walk past us.

"We got her fingernails," he said to me matter-of-factly in Spanish, looking over his shoulder, giving the bag a shake for emphasis, as he walked out of the front door. Deb and I looked at one another in utter disbelief and burst out laughing. *This cannot f-ing be happening,* I thought and we continued to laugh hysterically until tears streamed down our faces.

Cruz had moved out from behind his desk, to greet a gentleman wearing a white cotton shirt with a nametag affixed to the pocket, who had just walked through the door as Jorge Silva was walking out. They chatted for a minute in the middle of the lobby, looking over at the two of us every so often, like we were crazy. We probably looked crazy because we could not stop laughing.

The man with the nameplate approached us, and reintroduced himself. Deb and I were so caught up in our laughter, neither one of us had recognized him as the travel agent, Jesus, from the agency on the corner whom we had met briefly yesterday and had asked about translating for us. Jesus had come to the Ministerio to see if we still needed help, and Cruz told him there were still questions that he needed to ask us. Cruz led us back past the office of the DA, who I imagined was on his way back to the morgue—or somewhere—with his baggy of evidence, and Jesus asked which of us would like to be questioned first.

Debbie volunteered and followed the two men into the modest office. Left standing in the hallway to wait my turn, I paced back and forth, staring through the wire reinforced window, where Deb was instructed to sit in one of two office chairs facing the front of a plain grey metal desk. An older IBM typewriter sat on the return where the translator took his seat. Cruz stood leaning comfortably against a bank of filing cabinets across from where Debbie sat. I couldn't hear the questions he asked Deb, but saw the back of her head moving as she spoke and the translator typed out her responses.

Nervously anticipating my own turn in the hot seat, I walked down the hall for just a second and when I returned, I was shocked to see Cruz casually gripping the thick rubber handle of a very large knife in his right hand! *Oh my God! What the fuck do I do now?* I thought. Peering through the glass, paralyzed and frozen, I could feel my pulse in my throat and hear my own heartbeat ringing in my ears. I watched his mouth move, as he continued to question Debbie, slapping the flat smooth side of the long curved blade into the palm of his left hand, rhythmically, as though he had caught a beat.

My mouth went dry, and the choice to scream was not an option. Just as I was trying to formulate a plan for my next move, Debbie shot Cruz a look that I have seen on a few occasions: her "don't fuck with me" look with her eyes narrowed and her mouth tightened. Then she said a few words to the translator, and Cruz set the knife down. The interview lasted only a few minutes longer, and Debbie opened the office door to tell me it was my turn. We exchanged wide-eyed, knowing looks and she squeezed my arm as we passed through the doorway, trading places.

Still shaken and afraid to look Cruz directly in the face, I kept my eyes firmly planted on the pattern of the speckled, dirty linoleum floor, and I sat where Debbie had just been questioned. In the corner of the room, piled in a messy heap, a swatch of bright red fabric caught my eye and I shot to attention in my seat, stunned by what I saw.

"Puedo tocar la ropa? I stuttered, mouth agape, in disbelief. *Is that my mother's clothing?* "Can I touch it?" I asked quickly, standing, not waiting for his reply.

Cruz nodded, to me, but I was already hovering over the jumble of clothing, a blanket and what else, I could not yet tell. I knelt down and reached into the center of the swell of fabric for the red garment and pulled it free. I stood holding the shoulders of my mother's sweatshirt, the one she was last photographed in standing at the Wells Fargo ATM, making a deposit on the day she disappeared—and the one she had just died in. I examined the shirt, touching it's dusty polo collar and ran my hands over the body and arms, which were covered in straw-like brush and small dirty brown spots. I focused on the outline of my hands against the orange red fabric, and suddenly realized I had just placed my own fingerprints all over a piece of evidence in a murder investigation. *Oh dear God, what have I done?* I thought, dropping the garment back to the floor as if I had just learned it was covered in flesh-eating bacteria.

I could hardly concentrate on the questions I was being asked, because I so feared the unbelievable mistake I had just made, but I couldn't help myself; it was the last thing my mother wore, and I had to touch it. After my interview was concluded, Debbie and I were told the Ensenada investigative team had finished up with their work in Puertecitos and they would be in San Felipe soon.

★　　★　　★

When they arrived in a black suburban with tinted windows, I felt as though the Secret Service had just pulled in, but Deb and I very quickly learned that they were not necessarily in town to protect or to serve us. We were escorted to an office and the smaller gentleman from the group thankfully introduced himself in English. His name was Miguel Ortiz. He was dressed in jeans and a brown leather jacket, had a nice smile and kind eyes, and told Deb and me that he would be translating for us. The remaining detectives joined us in the office for introductions and the microscopic room began to feel quite claustrophobic when we realized that we were, in fact, considered suspects, as was everyone else in our family.

Mr. Ortiz introduced each of the men to Deb and me; then their questions began to ping pong back and forth across the room between detectives, the translator, and us for about twenty minutes. The biggest detective had a buzz cut and huge hands. I promptly christened him "Flatop" in my mind because it was easier to pronounce than his real name, Gerrardo, which could leave me tongue-tied trying to trill the r's. He asked, "Do you have a photograph of your mother with you?"

"No, we don't," I said, feeling a bit guilty for not having one in my purse, "but if you have Internet access, I can get one for you." I thought about how many times I had Googled Mom's name and the missing poster had come up.

The detectives spoke amongst themselves in Spanish and then to Cruz, and he told them there was an Internet café near the Ministerio.

"Will you go with the detectives now to a get a picture of your mother?" asked Miguel Ortiz.

"Yes, of course," I said, looking at Debbie, to see if she would be coming, too.

"I'll stay here and talk with your sister," Miguel said.

I'm not at all comfortable leaving Debbie or walking somewhere with these strangers, I thought, *but I have no choice."*

A burst of warm ocean air blew over me as the two large detectives held open the metal-framed glass doors for me to walk through. The streets were quiet in the neighborhood surrounding the Ministerio, and it had grown dark while Debbie and I were being questioned inside. I had a vague sense of the direction we were headed but waited to walk behind the two large detectives who seemed to be in charge. The remaining officers stepped in on either side of me—and suddenly I felt surrounded, conspicuous, and in trouble, as I caught the curious looks on the faces of people who passed our odd group on the street. I wished that Miguel Ortiz had come with us to translate, but he stayed behind with Debbie to continue to interview her further. I did not like being separated from Debbie; we had promised our family we would stay together. As we walked down the street, in order to break the ice, I asked each of the officers their names and they all kindly introduced themselves.

In the café Flattop spoke quickly to the manager, and the handful of customers who had been quietly typing away on the desktops were shuffled out of the building. The computers were lined up in a simple L shape against two walls. The detective pointed to a chair in the corner of the room and I took my seat. Flattop continued to speak to the owner while Espinoza and Morales assumed their places huddled behind me. The old cream-colored work station was filthy with the fingerprints of the customers who had sat there before me.

My hands, moist from the humidity, trembled as I reached to place them on the keyboard. I drew them back to my lap for a moment, wiping the sweat from my palms on the thighs of my jeans and began to type. I knew that I could find a news article, video, or Mom's "missing" poster if I searched. I had done that exact thing many times in the previous week on my laptop at home in the hope of finding new information or theories about Mom's whereabouts, and to read articles and review the videos of interviews my sisters and I had conducted. I nervously typed in "Jane Kling" and nothing came up.

I felt the herd behind me stir with anticipation and impatience, so I typed "Vista, California" into the search criteria and several results popped up. Reaching for the mouse, I moved the blinking arrow over the word "missing," and clicked. The image of Mom's smiling face filled the screen, my chin dropped to my chest and I closed my eyes, slumping over to cry. I felt the breath of all three detectives as they leaned in over me to get a closer look at the monitor. Wiping my face with the back of my hand, I turned to the detective on my left.

He bowed his head a bit to look into my puffy wet eyes, "Es su madre?" he asked timidly.

It took me a minute to respond to his simple question: "Is this your mother?" I stared at him blankly as I struggled with the simple translation for the words floating in my brain. The obvious answer was yes, but my first thought was to say, "Fue mi madre." "*That* was *my mom,*" I said, numbly, with tears streaming down my chin.

Flattop instructed the store manager to print a copy of Mom's picture and we walked in silence down the dark streets back to the Ministerio where Debbie was speaking with Miguel Ortiz. The lobby was now significantly more crowded than when I had left about a half hour earlier. I followed the detectives back to the office area where Deb was waiting for me. She told me that the people in the lobby were all brought in for questioning by Miguel Ortiz and Alejandro Morales, and that there was someone who had been at the scene when Mom's body was discovered, who wanted to speak with us. As we followed Miguel towards the lobby, a loud cat-call screeched down the hall in our direction, sending me nearly out of my skin. Lying on the floor of a small, closet-sized jail cell a few feet away, an apparently drunk jailbird mumbled out Spanish profanities as we passed.

In the lobby we were introduced to a slight gentleman with a thin mustache who greeted us in decent English. Cesar, the pastor from a church in Puertecitos, told Deb and me how sorry he was about our mother, and that he had stayed with her body until the authorities came to take her away in the night because he worried that the packs of coyotes that roam in the area might consume her remains.

He explained that a young brother and sister, the children of the owner of the campo where Mom was found, had happened upon Mom's body while out hunting for octopus, and at the same time, an American woman's adult daughter and boyfriend had arrived there. *That must be the woman who took the pictures of Mom's body and sold them to Channel 8,* I thought. Authorities were phoned and Cesar heard the call on his radio. I thanked Cesar for protecting our mother's body, and realized just how lucky we were to have found her at all.

Feeling a bit safer with the posse of detectives from Ensenada in town and probably too exhausted to know better, Deb and I walked back to the Hacienda Don Jesus in the dark that night—we were beginning to feel like regulars.

★   ★   ★

The next day, intent on leaving San Felipe as soon as possible, we focused on the important task at hand: we wanted to know when we could take Mom's body home and what needed to be done to make that happen. In addition to wanting the body for the memorial, we also wanted a second autopsy in the US. We met with Miguel Ortiz first thing. "We were wondering about taking our mom's body home for a second autopsy. Can you help us get that done?" I asked.

"You can't take an unembalmed body across the border," Ortiz said, "and your mother's body is filled with sawdust anyway; there would be nothing for them to examine."

Debbie and I looked at each other in dismay for what felt like the hundredth time on this debacle of a trip, and we were both at the breaking point. We had imagined and seen every awful thing about our mother's body, but the latest revelation—that she was filled with sawdust—gave me visions of Mom's body, Frankenstein-like and pieced back together. I closed my eyes and willed the image from my thoughts.

"So what is our choice here, Miguel?" Deb asked.

"You can have her cremated here in Mexico," he said.

"We have to call our sisters first; we won't make a decision like that without them," I said, frustrated that there were no other choices for us.

Deb and I stepped outside and dialed Sherri. She and Kim were together at Mom's house starting work on a video and the program for the memorial. Debbie reviewed what Miguel had just told us about Mom's body, and we all agreed that having Mom cremated was probably best for two reasons: there was no logical place for her to be buried, and we could spread her ashes someplace that would have made her happy.

We were so ready to leave San Felipe. Deb and I ran into town and hit every ATM we could find to gather enough cash to pay the coroner to release Mom's body to Mexicali for cremation. Our second stop was at a small travel agency to figure out how to get a ride to the Mexicali/Calexico border crossing where Rick would pick us up later that night. The gentleman informed Debbie and me that our best bet was a taxicab, and they would only accept cash, which made us both nearly burst out laughing. We had just collected all the cash we could get a hold of to pay the coroner.

"How much is that going to cost us?" Deb asked.

"Three hundred dollars," he replied.

We looked at each other for a split second, and Debbie's expression told me she would have given a limb to get the hell out of Mexico at that very moment. We nodded "yes" at the same time.

Deb and I had one more stop before we returned to the Ministerio to meet with the coroner Pablo Meza to pay him for the release of Mom's body to Mexicali for cremation. We went to Sagrado Corazon, the pharmacy where our translator, Octavio worked to say goodbye and thank him for his help. We also wanted to ask him about the drugs that are sold in Mexico available for purchase without a prescription. Debbie told me about how Mom had done this in the past, buying everything from antibiotics to estrogen, and we thought that maybe she had come to San Felipe to stock up on Tamiflu or Soma for herself or to sell for profit.

Deb pushed the glass door open ahead of me, and I followed her to the counter, where we were greeted by the saleswoman.

"Hola!"

"Hola. Esta trabajando Octavio, ahora?" *Is Octavia working now?*

"No, el esta en Puertecitos, hoy." *No, he is in Puertecitos, today.*

"Como?" *What?* I asked dumbfounded.

"El va a regresar a San Felipe manana." *He is going to return to San Felipe tomorrow.*

"Muchas gracias, hasta luego." I said, grabbing Debbie by the elbow to lead her away from the counter.

"Did you get that?" I said, pushing us both towards the door. "Octavio is in Puertecitos." I whispered in her ear, as we stepped through the door onto the dirty sidewalk, then broke into conversation when the door closed behind us. We had been with Octavio on two separate occasions discussing the fact that Mom's body was found in Puertecitos, and he had not once mentioned any knowledge of the area. Had Octavio been in the Ministerio to insinuate himself into the case to find out what authorities knew because he or someone he knew had something to do with Mom's murder? Deb and I felt like naive idiots to have trusted a perfect stranger. From that point on, everyone in Mexico was a suspect until proven otherwise.

Deb and I jumped into the cab for our ride to the border, completely fatigued and melancholy. We had to leave Mom behind, and somewhere in Mexico, our mother's body would soon be turned to ash.

EIGHT

The Investigation

I was thankful to be back home where everything was familiar—my family, my friends, my dog, and my house. But when I was greeted by Clark and Katy, who sweetly hugged me around the waist, their scent filled me at once with both relief and sadness as their probing, stricken eyes looked to me for reassurance. I knew then, that for me, nothing would feel the same again. I wouldn't shake off what I had experienced in Mexico. I wouldn't erase what I had seen. Life as I knew it was completely changed.

That first night home, I fell into bed exhausted and speechless. There was too much to tell and no energy to tell it. Although I had fallen asleep quickly, I remained asleep for only a few hours. Startled awake by the image of Debbie and me as we stood over Mom's body just before Pablo Meza pulled back the sheet to reveal Mom's face, I forced my eyes open. I was tangled up in my comforter, as if I had been wrestling someone in my sleep. I threw the covers off and headed downstairs. Bailey followed me down to the family room couch and sat next to me while I cried hysterically, and he gently licked my hands when I wiped my tears. My mind raced from thought to thought, *Who did this? Why did they do it? And where are they now?* Eventually, too tired to think anymore, I fell back to sleep around 4:00 am with Bailey curled up next to me.

I woke a few hours later and walked straight to the coffee maker to grab my first cup. I felt like I had been on the losing end of a street fight, and it was going to be a really long day. Grabbing one of Katy's notebooks from the counter, I sat down at my kitchen table and wrote out a list of all the tasks I needed to accomplish in the next week, before the memorial. Getting Mom's ashes back to the United States was near the top of the list, but Clark and Katy were my first concern. Rick had offered to take them to school that morning, and as soon they were out the door, I placed a call to Tim Reese, the principal at the middle school, to inform him that the kid's were dealing with the murder of their grandmother and to express my concerns about the media. The news of Mom's murder was being plastered all over San Diego county, and after Channel 8 released the Karla Nelson photos against my wishes, I worried that reporters might be bold enough to come to Mission Viejo to ask questions or shoot video. I wouldn't put it past them to show up unannounced at my children's school.

"Mrs. Taylor, I am so sorry about your mother," Tim said. "I live in Oceanside and have been following the television coverage since she went missing."

"Thank you," I said, surprised that he knew about Mom's death but touched by his kindness. "Could you please inform Clark and Katy's teachers of the situation. I hope they will be sympathetic and look out for my kids during school hours."

"Of course," he said, "I will."

I felt better after making the call, but I hadn't dared to say what I was really afraid of. I was scared out of my skin about a killer who hadn't been caught yet coming to Orange County.

The following morning, after school drop off, I met a handful of my closest girlfriends at the local coffee shop to tell them about Mom's murder and my trip to Mexico. I wanted to tell them all at once, because I didn't have the energy to repeat the story several times. Saying it out loud and seeing the sad looks on my friend's faces made the whole nightmare real, even though it felt like I was still dreaming. It felt like the more people who knew about Mom's murder, the more real it got—no more denial. The girls sweetly asked what they could do to help and I told them that there wasn't really anything I could think of. I was just focused on planning the memorial and getting Mom's ashes back.

I was running out of time, though. Mom's memorial service was in four days, and I was really stressing out. Sher had asked me to speak with the funeral home in Mexicali where Mom was to be cremated to coordinate the pick-up of her remains at the border. I called right away, and the director told me his facility had not yet received Mom's body from San Felipe. And to complicate matters further, he told me there was additional paperwork and a large sum of money still owed for the transport of the body between San Felipe and Mexicali. Debbie and I believed we had already paid the coroner in San Felipe all the necessary fees, but it was too late. Mom's body would not be moved to Mexicali until the weekend. The cremation process took a period of time and the paperwork allowing us to bring the ashes into the United States had not been filed. It was clear that we would be forced to go ahead with the memorial without a body.

★   ★   ★

Standing in my closet on Monday morning, April 3, less than a week since Debbie and I had traveled to San Felipe to identify Mom's body, I pulled a black wrap dress over my head and hips, smoothed the wrinkles with my hands, zipped myself up, and slipped into my black patent leather pumps. I walked out of the closet over to the drawer and pulled out the smooth long strand of pearls that Rick had given me the first Christmas we were married.

I fastened the clasp and stepped in front of the bathroom mirror that hung above my sink to adjust the necklace. Although my eyelids were heavy and had dark circles under them from lack of sleep, I thought Mom would be proud of me today. My sisters and I had planned a service that would reflect the image that Mom wanted the world to see of her and her family.

Mom had always been obsessed with weight, her own and her children's. I always felt she was especially concerned with mine. My sisters and I often joked that we were weaned on diet soda and I, personally, had been introduced to every diet from Scarsdale to the Grapefruit diet by the time I was ten years old. I had been cursed with a boxy body shape, with thin legs, but thicker around the middle, and even on my best day it was difficult for me to cram into the narrow-waisted style of clothing that was popular when I was growing up. Mom would bring home clothes for Kim and me, and I could not quite understand why mine never fit. It wasn't until I was much older that I realized that Mom bought me the size of clothing she *wanted* me to be, not the size I actually was, and consequently, I always felt uncomfortable in my clothes and in my own skin.

But I had slimmed down in the last several months. Stress will do that to you. Now I was zipped comfortably into my size eight dress, a respectable "single digit" size, of which I felt confident she would have approved.

Mom also would have approved of the other aspects of the memorial and reception that had been planned in her honor. Sherri, Kimi, and Tiffany had secured a beautiful church, lovely music, and a simple program. Debbie asked Mike, Keith, and Rick to speak about Mom on our behalf, and I planned a beautiful reception at the local country club, complete with her favorite, fresh yellow roses on every table. The only thing missing was Mom.

Rick, Clark, Katy, and I drove together down the highway I had traversed back and forth so often over the last few weeks. When we pulled into the church parking lot, I was surprised to see two television news vans parked at the curb. We walked together down the center aisle of the church to take our seats, which was beginning to fill up quickly with family, friends, and co-workers, and I noticed the television cameras were tucked discreetly up above the main floor in the balcony. The simple white altar was covered in the gorgeous flowers that people had kindly sent, and Mom's smiling face glowed on a screen that looped video full of our family pictures and memories above it. We all sat in the church pew numb and crying, and most of the rest of the service was a complete blur to me.

When the service concluded, my sisters and I gathered at the back door of the church in a receiving line, lined up youngest to oldest, like we had every year for our Christmas picture. We thanked everyone who had come to pay their respects to Mom. It was comforting to have so many friends and family there to offer support, but I was struck with a peculiar feeling as I was introduced to stranger after stranger who had worked for or were friends of Mom's from Vista: I kept thinking that I might be shaking the hand of Mom's murderer. I acted gracious because I didn't want to be rude, but what I felt, overwhelmingly, was suspicious. A woman whom I had never met before, who resembled my mom with her petite build and short blond hair, came rushing up to me in the line and introduced herself.

"Hello, I'm Diana Stuart and your mom was my closest friend," she said, hugging me too tightly.

"Oh," I said, shocked because I had never even heard the woman's name before in my life. "I'm Lauri."

"This will be helpful to you and your sisters, make sure you share it with them later," she said, swiftly shoving a small envelope into my hand.

"I will," I said, lamely, placing it into my purse, and turned to introduce Ms. Stuart to Kim, who was standing next to me in line. *"Could she have information about Mom's death?"* I thought.

People continued to stream through one after another, offering their condolences, and many explaining how they knew Mom—*I was a customer at her store, I own the shop next to your mom's, I was your mom's cleaning lady, I worked for your mom at the big store.* I was relieved when I turned back to greet the next guest in line and was met with a hug and the sweet, comforting smile of my dear friend, Teresa. We chatted for just a minute, and while Teresa was hugging me one more time, I glanced around the room and was struck by how many people I didn't know. I had been so uninvolved in Mom's life when she died, that I had no idea who all these people were who claimed to have known her so well.

A few days after the memorial, Rick called to let me know that there was some good news regarding Mom's ashes: they would be at our house in Mission Viejo that afternoon. The weekend before the memorial, I had spoken with Michael Mathe, one of Rick's employees, who was in charge of the International division including Mexico and South America, because he was fluent in Spanish. I was so distraught and needed help anywhere I could get it.

I had asked Michael about helping communicate with the funeral home in Mexicali. Michael and his wife, Pam, had been on many dealer incentive trips with Rick and me over the years, and he had always been complimentary and supportive of my efforts to communicate with customers in Spanish. Michael called me to get the numbers for our contacts in Mexicali and San Felipe, and told me that a Toshiba dealer in Mexico had held a position in government in Baja and for me not to worry, because between the two of them, they would find a way to get Mom's ashes back for me. I would soon find out the heroic efforts Michael made to make good on his promise. Rick arrived home later that day gingerly carrying something tucked in a white plastic Hyatt hotel dry cleaning bag, and set it on the kitchen table.

"What in the world is that?" I asked.

"It's your mom's ashes," he said, almost apologetically, with a face that showed he felt awful that she hadn't arrived in something more grand.

"Oh," I said, a bit shocked. "How did Michael get this done?"

"You are not going to believe it," Rick said, shaking his head. "Michael and Carlos, my dealer in Mexico, paid the funeral home director off, since they didn't have any of the required paperwork. They smuggled your mom's ashes across the border. I met them at the hotel in Irvine and Michael felt bad about walking through the lobby to hand me the box uncovered so he grabbed this bag."

"Oh my God," I said, half laughing. *Would the bizarre stories never stop coming?*

★   ★   ★

There were a few more things to accomplish before my sisters and I could get back to a somewhat normal way of life—well normal, with the exception of an ongoing murder investigation. Mom's house needed to be packed up and her stores needed to be closed. Mom had no money, no assets, no retirement or savings, so everything had to be shut down. Disgruntled consignors showed up at A&J Consignment, one after another, looking for either the furniture they had consigned or for checks for their portion of the proceeds from the sale of their merchandise, and neither was there for them. Sherri and Adam, who were the most familiar with the day to day operations of the stores, were left to deal with the financial issues of the consignors and employees, which began to take it's toll.

The financial issue was causing some tension among the sisters because Debbie and I and our husbands didn't feel as though we were responsible for the liabilities of a business we hadn't agreed to support. Unlike Keith and Sherri, we had never invested in it. On a phone call to discuss the issue with Sherri and Keith, in a moment of high frustration, it was suggested to me that I had never been there for my mom financially or otherwise, which made my heart ache. I stood my ground about the business, but the insinuation hit me like a hammer between the eyes, and confirmed what my guilty conscience reminded me of daily.

My sisters and I were joined by family friends, who came to Vista to help pack up Mom's house. Dad even came back to town to help us with the final cleaning and return of the key to Mom's landlord. I had not spent much time in Mom's home in Vista, and everyone kept asking me what I wanted from the house. I chose a decorative box covered in fleurs de lis that Kim had suggested I might like when we had spent the night together in Mom's guestroom after Katy's birthday. Just as Mom was not married to her real estate, she was not married to, or sentimental about, her personal belongings. Mom always preferred brand new things or what appeared to be new, so she did not hang onto anything for very long.

There was one exception to that rule; she did hang on to her animals. Bear and Charlie had moped around the house for the last month. Everyone had done their best to give them love and attention, but they were as sad and confused as the rest of us. A decision had to be made about who would take the dogs. Kim had her beloved kitty, Jack, that Mom had given her just a year ago, and he was not fond of other kittens, and would certainly not take kindly to a one hundred-pound dog. I seemed like a logical choice because my love of dogs was on par with Mom's love of dogs, but

Bailey didn't mix well with other male dogs. Debbie and Sherri, who seemed to be carrying so much of the burden already, agreed to take the dogs. Big fluffy Bear would go to Debbie's house and Charlie boy would go with Sher to her new house.

It had been three weeks since Mom's memorial. We had heard nothing from law enforcement in Mexico or San Diego, but finally Burt Long phoned Deb to request that all of the sisters be present at a meeting with detectives from Mexico at SDSO Headquarters to update us on progress in Mom's investigation. At the memorial a reporter had casually mentioned to Rick that law enforcement in Mexico was tracking a male suspect to Mexico City. *Maybe we are meeting because they have caught the suspect from Mexico City,* I thought. I was thrilled to have the opportunity to meet with law enforcement and hopeful to hear that detectives had come up with some significant leads in three weeks.

I have never been in any real trouble in my life; in fact, the closest I had ever come to being in an actual police station occurred when I was a senior in high school. As part of a Kiwanis Club sponsored program, a group of students and I were given the privilege of choosing which honorary position in local government we would like to hold for the day. Like many of my contemporaries, I had grown up entranced by the cop shows of the late 70s: *Starsky & Hutch, Streets of San Francisco,* and *Chips,* with our local hometown hunk, Erik Estrada, in the lead. I loved them all, as a teenage girl would, but who I wanted to *be* was a cross between Angie Dickinson of *Police Woman* and Farrah Fawcett of *Charlie's Angels.* I wanted the gun, the badge, and the cool clothes, so I asked to be the police chief for the day. Despite my enthusiasm for the position, someone else, a boy, got the job and I was made the honorary fire captain instead.

This blow did not diminish my love of crime drama or my fascination with police work, forensics, and solving crimes, and now

I would be in a real police office, part of a real investigation—and, I feared, closer to real trouble than I wanted to be.

Deb, Kim, and I were asked to show our driver's licenses at the desk and given badges with our names printed just below the headline "Homicide Division." Sherri was closing escrow on her new house that afternoon and was disappointed she couldn't be there. Detective Long met us in the lobby, and we followed him to the conference room on the fourth floor. The room was packed, all men, and not one of them in the stylish uniforms my television idols had worn, but all in some variation of business casual: slacks, shirts, a few ties, and some sport coats. Deb and I recognized some of the detectives from Mexico and waved hello across the massive table. Flattop, the big guy who had walked me to the Internet café, smiled back, a bit uncomfortably. Miguel Ortiz was missing from the group and I wondered how the detectives would be communicating. Long asked Deb, Kim, and me to sit near the middle and on one side of the conference table, while practically everyone else took seats on the other side and at either end of the table. We were definitely sitting on an island alone.

Sgt. Lewis of SDSO, whom none of us had met before, introduced himself, and then went round the large table introducing each individual and their rank at SDSO or the agency they were associated with. The sergeant then turned over the meeting to the gentleman he had introduced as Eduardo Reyes, a Special Agent from the California Department of Justice, who, he explained, was there to translate for us. Eduardo sat dead center in the table between Mexican detectives and SDSO detectives, and his boss, Antonio Ruiz. His light hair, muscular build, and tan skin gave him the appearance of another Southern California raised detective. There was warmth and empathy in his eyes, I felt it, even before he spoke.

"I understand you speak Spanish?" he said, kindly, looking in my direction.

"Yes, I do," I answered.

Eduardo gently explained that the detective from Mexico would speak first, then he would translate for the group, and if we had any questions whatsoever to stop him anytime. I nervously moved my hand over the three pages of questions that I had printed out in the middle of the night, and nodded.

"The detectives from Ensenada have information they would like to share and would like to ask you some questions."

With Eduardo translating, we were told that authorities in Mexico believed Mom had been strangled by chokehold and tests had confirmed she was not sexually assaulted. They noted that there was a prescriptive level of a drug, possibly Soma, in her system, and that she showed signs of pulmonary edema. They asked about Mom's business, her relationship with employees, neighbors, and friends.

"What about your father? Where does he live?"

"He and Mom have been on friendly terms for years. He lives in northern California."

"What about your nephew, Adam, who quit his job before your mother disappeared? Where has he been?"

"Adam has been in Vista helping to run Mom's consignment stores the entire time since Mom went missing."

The questioning then shifted, and Eduardo explained to us that the detectives had brought a composite sketch that was drawn based on interviews with the staff at the Hotel Costa Azul in San Felipe. Statements from the front desk clerk and a security guard at the hotel led detectives to believe that Mom stayed there for the first few days she was in San Felipe. The female clerk had given them a very vivid description of their person of interest, but Mexican and US detectives could not determine the identity of the suspect. I was frozen with hope for just a moment, daydreaming. *They have a real suspect and maybe I will be the one to identify him,* I thought, feeling exhilarated and slightly relieved by the idea that this whole nightmare might end, if I could simply identify the suspect. *I need to be the one to fix this, so Mom will forgive me, so I can forgive myself for not being there for her,* I thought.

"Do you recognize this person?" Eduardo asked, sliding the paper across the smooth laminate in front of the three of us.

"It's a woman," he added, just as he stopped pushing and lifted his hand away.

Our heads snapped up, in unison, and we stared up at him, astonished.

"What?"

I had assumed the suspect was a man, and based on Deb and Kim's reactions, they had, too. The news media had reported about the pursuit of a male suspect in Mexico City and that was what Rick was told about at Mom's memorial. Deb, Kim, and I hovered closely, leaning in for a better look.

I sat back in my chair, shaking my head "no." I didn't have a clue who the very masculine, stocky woman, wearing a baseball cap and plaid shirt could be, and was disappointed that I had nothing to add.

"I think this looks like Sylvia Murphy," Debbie said, holding the corner of the paper, tipping it in Kim's direction.

Mom's cleaning lady? I thought, watching Kim take a closer look.

"Yeah, I do, too," Kim said. "She has the same shape face."

And, just like that, I was out of the loop. I could barely remember what Mom's cleaning lady looked like, and consequently, had zero to offer to the current discussion. I knew I had met her briefly at the memorial, because Kim reminded me about it. In my silence, I thought about how truly disconnected Mom and I had been when she died. I did not know her friends or her co-wokers, and they all seemed to know my mother better than I did. Trying to focus my attention on the list of questions in front of me, I wondered if anyone could see the shame and guilt that devoured me. I kept my eyes glued to my paper.

"Can we get Sherri and Adam to take a look?" Debbie asked the detective.

The detectives conferred with one another and the composite sketch was faxed to Sherri and Adam. A follow up call to Sherri confirmed that she saw a resemblance, as well. A flurry of questions about Sylvia Murphy followed, none of which I could answer—where did she live? How long had she worked for Mom? Was she married? Then the tone of questioning shifted in a way that shocked us all.

"Is it possible your mom was in a relationship with a woman?"

We all looked at each other completely puzzled.

"Our Mother was married four times," Debbie offered.

"She loved men," Kim bolstered.

"Your mother had tattoos; they appeared to be sexual—roses and leaves . . ."

There it was, their suspicion, dangling out there—*they think Mom was in a lesbian relationship that went sour.* Now at least we knew what they were thinking, but I wasn't prepared to deal with any more revelations about Mom, regardless of whether they were true or not, and I charged into my instinctive "protect image" mode.

"Mom had girlfriends she traveled with her whole life, and we have four girls in the family. It was not unusual for all of us to pile into a room together," I said, shifting uncomfortably in my seat, the expressionless faces of the Mexican detectives indicating to me that they were not really buying my explanation.

As worthy of note to me, though, were the expressions of US law enforcement. *Are they really rolling their eyes?* I thought, feeling uneasy about the odd dynamic in the room—not because I thought they were rolling their eyes at our answers, but because they were showing obvious disrespect for the opinions and line of questioning coming from Mexico. Embarrassed by Detective Long's immature posture and body language, I adjusted my own to be more attentive and focused on their presentation, sitting up straighter in my seat. I did not want to offend these detectives in any way whatsoever. The detectives from Ensenada were in charge of my mother's murder investigation and I felt like any answers about Mom's death were coming through them.

When all the questions in the room had been answered, Eduardo Reyes focused on Deb, Kim, and me.

"Please take my card," he said, sliding three business cards across the table to us. "If you have any questions, feel free to call me."

"Thank you so much for your help today," I said, leaning across the table to shake his hand.

"My pleasure," he said smiling, the corners of his eyes softening. "And I mean it about calling . . . don't hesitate," he said, with a wink.

I had not had much interaction with Burt Long, but the vibe of arrogance that he emitted told me he would not be someone I could call for any reason. My gut told me that Eduardo was sincere and if I needed help, I would feel perfectly comfortable calling him.

I left our first investigative meeting feeling completely flustered by the experience. I had hoped for a miracle, a case that was swiftly wrapped up, the news of an arrest delivered to our family, just as I had seen my favorite characters do so many times on my favorite shows. But my shows and the characters were fiction, and what my family was living was brutally real. I wished I could change the channel or turn the show off all together, but I couldn't. My guilt wouldn't let me—not until I knew the truth.

NINE

❦

Therapy

The noise from the television had become the bane of my existence. It could make my skin crawl, my scalp tingle, my throat close, my heart race, and my stomach heave, depending on which particular show was on at the time. It often sent me out of the room in a flash or straight to my knees in tears. The volume alone, if notched one click too high, agitated me as though I had just downed two Venti French Roasts from Starbucks on an empty stomach. Fight scenes were particularly disturbing. The sound of flesh hitting flesh was unbearable and only served to add audio to the video that played in my dreams at night.

I couldn't fall asleep at all, let alone while the television roared in the background. I began sleeping, for the few hours that I managed to string together, with my head sandwiched firmly between two pillows to muffle the noise from the TV.

"Do you want me to turn off the TV," Rick asked nearly every night for a week.

"No, I'm fine," I would insist, burying my head, soaking my pillow with tears, hoping that if I said it, it would be true. I tried to pretend that everything was okay, that I was okay, but I was doing a crappy job. I felt like my time was running out on not being okay. How long could I go on being sad, sleepless, distraught, and forgetful?

During the day when my family was out of the house, I did what I could to maintain the silence around me. My nerves could not take it any other way, and I believed that I could concentrate and focus better without the distraction of TV, radio, or music. The reality was I couldn't concentrate to save my life, except for when it came to the very precise details of my mother's case. Quite frequently, I would find myself in a room, wondering why I was there. I had become ridiculously hyper-focused on the specifics of the murder investigation, having proudly memorized every name, date, time, and relevant fact, but I struggled to remember the basic responsibilities of my own life, leaving dry cleaning when it was critical that it be picked up for my husband's impending business trip, or stranding a kid without lunch when I promised to bring one because the refrigerator was empty. But people were starting to lose their patience with me.

"Just pay the fucking bills," Rick barked in my direction after going through a stack of mail that lay unopened on the kitchen island one evening, the string of late notices strewn about in front of him. I cringed, but at that moment, I couldn't have cared less about the bills. I was completely numb and promptly set our utilities up on auto-pay so I didn't have to think about them or hear about them any longer. I burned with shame for letting my responsibilities go, but resentment began to boil in me as well because I felt so misunderstood. Lacking the strength to explain or defend myself, I turned inward and grew more and more silent at home.

In the morning after I got the kids off to school, the television and any other noise-producing apparatus were turned off and the house was quiet, but never quiet enough or quite possibly too quiet. I could not turn off the stream of thoughts and images that plowed through my brain. Everything in my world became a potential clue or sign. I could not get away from the visions of Mom in her final moments of terror, no matter how loud or how silent my environment became.

I had a tight supportive group of friends who generously listened to me when I could speak, indulged me in my silence when I could not, and gently prodded me out of isolation when I had disappeared for too long. We gathered for coffee, "Crazy Chicken" lunches, or a glass of wine in between running our kids to school, sports, and other activities. But even some of my oldest friendships became strained that summer because I was no longer equipped to handle even the slightest bit of dissention and began to act out of character.

Because our friend Sue was a trainer, we often spent time together exercising in the neighborhood. I knew intuitively that the fresh air, exercise, and good company were not only good for me but necessary to my well being. We walked the hills together, choosing the steepest inclines to get our heart rates up, then returned to Sue's driveway where she led a mini boot camp. Sue and I quickly discovered we actually enjoyed sweating and regularly chatted our way through difficult workouts.

Sue explained to me that her mother, Patricia, had died just two years earlier, without warning. Pat was a nurse, had raised five kids, and lived her life without major health issues. She went to the hospital for what was supposed to be a simple procedure and never left. It was completely devastating to Sue, and she generously and honestly shared with me how difficult grieving her mother's death had been. Sue spent much of the summer of Pat's death in bed, immobilized by her staggering grief. Two and a half years later, she still carried the shame over her inability to simply "snap out of it." Until that moment, I had no idea what grief was or how it could so wickedly consume your entire life. I was relieved to have such a close friend who could relate to what I was experiencing without judgment or comparison.

★   ★   ★

May of 2006 was a particularly difficult and emotional month with Mother's Day and Mom's birthday, May 22, falling within weeks of each other. Every holiday from now on would be a milestone, marked with the designation of the anniversary since Mom's murder: first Easter, first Birthday, and so forth. The thought of counting each holiday in this manner was heartbreaking and a devastating reminder that we still had no answers in the investigation. One afternoon while idling in the turn lane a few blocks from home and enjoying the quiet solitude of my car, I daydreamed for a moment and spoke to Mom as I did frequently when I was alone and missed her.

I promise I will find the person that did this to you and make you proud of me, again. I will do it to honor your memory and all that you taught me. Something good will come from this dreadful place . . . it has to.

Suddenly, a fire engine that had been sitting behind me at the light turned on its siren and the abrupt deafening shriek nearly sent me through the roof of my car. I began to cry hysterically, paralyzed for a moment, shaking violently as I gripped the steering wheel. I had hesitated just long enough that the frustrated fireman laid on the horn of his massive truck, which nearly caused me to vomit. Knees buckled, I pressed the gas, my car lurched forward, and and I pulled over to the curb as quickly as I could, collapsing onto my steering wheel in a blubbering heap.

By June it became more and more difficult for me to pretend that I felt okay. I was ultra sensitive, and I had zero patience. In line at the grocery store, mere acquaintances would tell me that my mother was in a better place and all that my family was going through was part of God's plan. I knew they didn't have any idea what to say to me, and that their intentions were sincere, because I had stood in their shoes before at funerals where I would struggle to come up with the perfect, comforting thing to say.

So when people tried to comfort me. I would bite my tongue and smile, but I would be thinking to myself, *Are you fucking kidding me? How could it possibly be God's plan for my Mom to die at the hands of a crazed killer in a barren desert wash and for someone else's mother to die peacefully in bed with their loving family gathered around holding her hand to usher her straight to heaven? Where is God now? Is there a God? What have I done to deserve this?*

My desire to protect myself from people's interest, comments, and advice extended from the grocery store to our social network. I couldn't motivate myself to go anywhere where people actually knew me, except for being with my girlfriends, where I felt safe to laugh or cry. Although we had a close circle of work friends, I stopped attending my husband's work functions and turned down the chance to go on his incentive trips, because I had lived with the self-imposed expectation that I had to maintain a certain image and that being truly authentic would be a violation of my duty as the boss' wife. Despite the guilt I felt about not doing "my job," I simply didn't have the strength to put on the entertainer's mask. I could not pretend to be the happy, interested, and engaging wife of the CEO. I had left her at the border and was hopeless that she was ever coming back.

Other issues prevented me from leaving town, as well. Once a total lover of travel and a confident flyer, I had become extremely fearful of getting on a plane. I was afraid of leaving my children at home because there was still a murderer on the lose, and I didn't want to miss a meeting or be out of touch in case something developed in the investigation. Worn down by truly kind people asking me how I was holding up or questions about the investigation that I did not have answers for, I began to isolate myself even more.

Growing up, Mom had instilled in all of us the "fake it 'til you make it" mentality, because no one, least of all her, wanted to see us unhappy, hear us cry or whine, or be any trouble whatsoever, for that matter. We were a well-oiled army, the five of us, following orders and preserving the sacred image of our happy, successful family. Even on those mornings after the house had erupted in violent arguments late into the night, warranting a visit from the local policeman to settle things down, we were expected to pack our lunches, march off to school, and make the honor roll. Anything short of strict adherence to the rules was seen as abhorrent and selfish.

I tried vehemently to follow the rules, live up to the standard and pretend like I wasn't scared or sad or sick, but it was an impossible standard for a nine-year-old or anyone else to live up to, and consequently, I was labeled the sensitive one, the one who cried too quickly and too often, who wet the bed (an awful inconvenience, not to mention downright humiliating) and always had a brutal sore throat. But even I began to master the skills of pretending as I got older—crying alone, if I had to, sobbing out my fears and frustration onto the fur of the closest stuffed animal or current pet. Occasionally, though, my face or my eyes would give me away.

"What's wrong with you?" Mom would ask.

"Nothing, I'm fine, I'm fine," I would chirp reassuringly, knowing she did not want to hear whatever my truth was. I'd shake my head for emphasis and swallow the emotion that enveloped me and dutifully plaster a smile on my face.

"I'm fine, I'm fine, I'm fine" became my mantra in the months following Mom's death, too. I would chant it silently in my head when I felt sick to my stomach with anxiety or fear, to relax and help myself fall asleep, or to hold back the tears that seemed to want to fall all the time now. But I was not convincing myself, and I woke up in early July 2006 at what felt like the bottom of the Grand Canyon. The fog of grief and shock that had protected me for the first few months following Mom's death had blinded me to the edge of the cliff, and I free-fell into the depths of despair. I opened my eyes that morning and panic washed over me. My heart raced and all I wanted was a pill or to be put to sleep until the nightmare was over.

I called Sue because she had casually mentioned to me that she had recently reconnected with a friend from middle school who was a therapist in our town. I was afraid to admit I needed help and deeply embarrassed because I had avoided therapy my whole life. But the truth of the matter was, I probably had needed therapy for most of my life. Sue gently reassured me and forwarded the contact information. I called immediately. I could not get to the therapist fast enough. I could not live this way, pretending I was okay, for even one more day.

★　　★　　★

The office was in a small stucco compound of mostly medical offices. The name on the nameplate read Dr. Elizabeth Bryant, PhD. I stepped through the door towards the sliding-glass window that divided the office from the waiting room. Soft music played from a small boom box on a table in the corner. Mercifully, there was no one else waiting, or I might have turned around and walked out the door right then. Two small leather sofas faced each other with a glass and iron coffee table between them, covered in women's magazines. I sat down.

A moment later, Dr. Bryant opened the hallway door and invited me to follow her down the hall to her office.

"Come on in. Can I get you a cup of tea?" she asked me, ges-
turing towards a long, cream leather sofa, where she wanted me
to sit.

"No, thank you, I'm fine," I said, surveying the titles of psychology books that lined the tall bookcase next to her desk.

She placed her cup of tea on the coffee table in front of us and
sat in the matching cream leather chair next to me.

"Tell me what brings you here," she said leaning back into the
chair, casually crossing her legs.

I took a deep breath and gave her the Cliff Notes version of
what had happened to Mom and our family since March, and
shared with her how I had been feeling.

"It is like I am having some sort of sympathetic reaction to
my mother being strangled; I often feel like I am suffocating and
can't catch my breath. My stomach is in knots constantly and I can
hardly swallow. The only thing I can really manage to get down
without feeling like I am going to choke is a spoonful of yogurt at
a time. I'm not sleeping much because I am awakened every night
about one in the morning by my nightmares. From about one to
four a.m., I sit downstairs in the family room with my dog, Bailey,
and cry. It is safe to cry then, because my kids don't see how sad I
really am, and maybe they won't see that I am falling apart. It feels
as though my whole world has imploded and nothing will ever be
the same. I will never be the same, but everyone expects me to be.
Can you give me something, a pill, anything to make this feeling
go away?"

The doctor gently clarified that she was not a medical doctor, but a psychologist and licensed marriage and family therapist,
so she could not prescribe medicine but she would refer me to
someone who could. My heart sank because it had taken every
ounce of guts I had to walk through her door in the first place

and the thought of having to tell my story someplace else, even to another doctor, felt completely overwhelming. She also told me that I could be suffering from some post-traumatic stress, based on the symptoms I had described. I crumpled and began to cry.

"What are you thinking about right now?" she asked softly, handing me a box of tissues.

"The last time I saw my mom," I squeaked, wiping my nose.

"It was December 11, 2005. As a Christmas present to Mom, my daughter, my sisters, and I took her to see a local production of *Cats*. She loved the music and she loved the kitties. When the show was over we got in separate cars to meet at a restaurant in my hometown, Manhattan Beach. Debbie, my eldest sister warned us that it would be difficult to find parking because the annual fireworks and pier Christmas lighting were happening downtown. It was a Sunday night and Katy had school in the morning, so after an hour of driving around, still without finding a place to park, we called and told the girls we would not be joining them for dinner and drove home to Orange County. I left my mom in the parking lot of the theatre that day thinking I would see her in a few minutes, but I never saw her again, never gave her another hug . . . never said goodbye."

"You didn't speak to your mom between December and March?" the Dr. asked cautiously, sipping from her teacup.

I felt my stomach turn, the guilt and shame instantly consuming me. I sucked in a large breath of air and swallowed hard.

"We had a difficult relationship," I said, looking down at my hands. "I loved my mom, but we were not close when she died." I had barely spoken the words before the tears began to pour out once again, soaking the chest of my shirt.

The hour had passed at lightning speed and I actually felt a little better when it was over. It was freeing to talk with someone who did not have preconceived notions about me or my mom, and who validated what I was experiencing. We made an appointment to see each other in a week and I silently hoped I could make it that long. All the way home, and all that night, I chanted, "*I'm fine, I'm fine, I'm fine.*"

TEN

ॐॐ

Lost Summer

I could not believe how quickly the summer was flying by but how slowly Mom's case progressed. Things had virtually slowed to a halt. The majority of my weekly therapy sessions were spent updating my therapist about insignificant developments in the case and venting my frustrations and fears about never finding any answers about Mom's death. Very little time was spent talking through my grief and feelings of isolation. How could Mom's killer be found if no one wanted to investigate? It was clear to me that SDSO had no interest in working with Mexico or with the family.

Our International liaison, Oscar Rivera, who worked for SDSO was nearly non-responsive to my calls and emails, and he carried the jaded attitude of someone who had had little success in solving cases like Mom's. He was kind and sympathetic enough, but he lacked enthusiasm for the work. It was a numbers game in Homicide. For every day that passed since Mom's murder, the likelihood of solving her case was exponentially reduced as new case files piled up on overworked detectives desks. It was a reality I clearly understood, but I was unwilling to accept because we weren't talking about a stranger. We were talking about my mother.

There had been little communication from SDSO following our meeting in May, so by early July my frustration over the case, coupled with my mounting anxiety, pushed me to pick up the phone. I needed some answers. Because of his work across the border, Oscar Rivera rarely answered, so I left a message asking him to return my call. Then I placed my next call to Detective Long.

He wasn't exactly sure who I was, until prompted, and put me on hold while he went to get the case file. "Can you tell me what day Sylvia Murphy was interviewed?" I asked.

"Ms. Murphy was interviewed on the 23rd of March, and there were no hits on her vehicle in or out of Mexico," he added—a little smugly, I thought.

"You seem somewhat unconvinced about Sylvia as a suspect," I said. "Do you have a theory?" I was done being nice. I wanted some answers.

"Well, I think the crime was committed by a Mexican, and I wish their detectives would concentrate on the scene. Your mother's body was found 100 yards from her vehicle and no one saw anything in broad daylight? It makes me think there was a cop involved. They didn't even allow us to process your mom's van . . . they just left me hanging," he said, referring to the detectives from Ensenada.

Detective Long's mistrust and repugnance for Mexican law enforcement were palpable, oozing through the phone line, covering me in a layer of contempt. At our first meeting in April, I had seen members of the SDSO Homicide unit, including, Burt Long, roll their eyes at comments made by the detectives from Ensenada, but at the time, I did not understand the reason for their impertinence and was personally embarrassed by the lack of respect they showed their Mexican counterparts. Now it made sense to me. The Mexican professionals had pissed off Detective Long early in the case, and he was unwilling to work with them. I pressed forward with my questions.

"I was wondering if you could coordinate a meeting with the detectives from Mexico, Eduardo Reyes, and possibly Agent Vincente from the FBI? It's been a few months since we have all gathered and I don't want to lose momentum in the case."

"I can provide a room for you to meet in, but you'll have to contact the detectives in Baja directly or through Oscar Rivera."

Wow, a room, how generous of him, I thought, stunned for a moment by his response. *He is the lead detective on my mother's murder investigation and all he can do for us is provide a room?* I remember having the clear and distinct thought: *I'm going to solve this case myself!*

"Uh, ok, I guess I'll do that," I blurted out and hung up the phone, nearly crushing the off button on my cell with my thumb. I felt my cheeks begin to burn with anger. *How dare he let his ego get in the way of doing his job properly on our case,* I thought. *He will not get away with this,* I began to formulate my next move, while one persistent thought began to buzz in my brain: *I am going to make you proud Mom, I promise.*

I had learned a fair bit about working with law enforcement in the last six months, but I needed help and advice from someone "in the business" whom I trusted had my family's best interest at heart. Eduardo Reyes, Special Agent with the California Department of Justice, was our guy.

Since our introduction at the initial meeting with SDSO in April, Eduardo had been a rock of encouragement and support for me, returning my calls promptly, or if he was unable to do so, he always offered a sincere apology and an explanation. The work he did everyday as a DOJ Special Agent was dangerous and top secret. If Eduardo was "out of the office," that was code for being in Mexico to handle something big, like a murder or child abduction. Eduardo was as close to a superhero as I was ever likely to have work on Mom's case, but what made him so endearing was his modesty about his job and his generosity with his time and patience for my questions. Previously, I had tried hard not to bother Eduardo too much, but something had changed in me and I needed his help. Eduardo would be my next call.

I helped Clark get packed up for Stanford Golf camp and drove him to catch his plane to San Francisco. I was grateful that he had plans to do something fun and exciting, but my anxiety amped up as I kissed him good-bye at bag check. I kept wanting to hug him one more time, and when he finally walked away, it was all I could do to get to the car without crying. Sliding into the seat, I buckled myself in and let the tears wash down my cheeks. *Please let him be safe*, I thought, begging the universe, crying harder as fear and anxiety choked me.

I was completely distraught when I was told that my mom had been murdered, but one of the first things that came to mind in that moment, besides my fear of being blamed for her death, was that I had avoided the worst tragedy of all—losing a child. In the great hunt for blessings that happens in the aftermath of the tornado of tragedy, when it felt as though my life was in ruin.

I was thankful, immensely thankful, that my children were okay. I grabbed a piece of clothing out of the dry cleaning pile that lay on the floor of the backseat of my car and wiped my face before pulling away from my parking spot.

Driving down the freeway towards home, still thinking about Clark on the airplane, I dialed Eduardo. As promised, and as he always seemed to do for me, he answered my call and kindly listened to me lament about Burt Long's bad attitude regarding the Mexican investigators, and about Sylvia Murphy as a suspect, and the general lack of effort on our case. I told him that our family was not asking for much. We simply wanted SDSO to conduct a proper investigation and rule out Sylvia Murphy as a suspect. Eduardo agreed that my expectations were not outlandish and recounted the fine points of a personal trip he had recently taken to San Felipe that he believed I might find interesting. Eduardo told me that he and some buddies had gone there to ride motorcycles and for some R&R.

"We stayed at a small hotel outside of town, just off the road you would take to get to Puertecitos. My friends and I were soaking in the pool after a long ride, having some beers, when I struck up a conversation with the hotel owner. He was from Long Beach, but had been living primarily in Mexico the last several years. I asked him if he had heard anything in town about your mother's murder. He became very animated and described to me that he had never seen anything like it before in Baja. Four detectives from Ensenada came to the hotel and basically "shook him down" for information about your mom. They asked to see his records, which he said had never happened in all the years he had been there."

"I wanted to tell you that story so you will trust your gut on these detectives. Although they don't have the training or resources we have in the States, they have been investigating, and they want to solve this case for your family. And the stuff with SDSO," he said, and then he paused. "Well, sometimes even the best investigators get stuck on one track in a case and work only to prove that theory. The trick, though, is being open to every possibility, which is a lot harder than you think."

My resolve to contact the Mexican authorities and get some of the men together "in a room" was now even stronger. Maybe all that was needed to solve this case was a little pressure. Maybe all that was needed was me to do the pressuring.

"That means a lot to me Eduardo, thank you. I'll call to check in with Miguel Ortiz and find out what is happening in the case on his side of the border line."

Miguel Ortiz and I had exchanged emails and occasional cell phone calls over the last few months, and I began to feel a comfort level conversing with him in our combined Spanish English language. I did not always understand what he was trying to convey to me, and he did not always understand what I was trying to convey to him, but we did our best and bonded over the imperfection of mastering the other's language. His kind emails were always laced with misspelled words and an endearing, but totally unnecessary apology for them. I became increasingly comfortable with our communication because Miguel had shown his honorable intentions over time.

He told me that there was a lot of pressure on their office to solve Mom's case and that up until recently, he had been fielding calls from the media and there had been interest in a movie. He reiterated Mexico's position about Sylvia Murphy: she was still the lead suspect because their investigators could not set aside the fact that when he, Velez, and Espinoza had shown up with Oscar Rivera to interview Sylvia back in May, she not only closely resembled the composite sketch but she was also wearing a plaid shirt that was strikingly similar to the one worn by the woman in the composite.

Miguel Ortiz had repeatedly asked SDSO for pictures of Sylvia Murphy so detectives could use them during questioning in San Felipe. SDSO was not only unresponsive to the family but to Mexican investigators, as well, and Miguel finally asked me directly if I could help them get surveillance photos of Sylvia. My sisters and I agreed we would help Ortiz, Velez, and Espinoza by paying to have the photos taken, because it appeared they were the only ones trying to investigate Mom's case.

Supporting their efforts was a huge step in gaining the trust of Miguel Ortiz and the PGJE, and this changed the way we interacted going forward. Miguel showed just how deep his suspicion of Sylvia ran, and how his trust of me had grown, on one memorable phone call. He asked if my family and I would be willing to participate in a ruse to get Sylvia across the border to Ensenada for questioning. I told him we would not, but we would help in any other way we could. Instead, we paid Chris Mendoza to spend a day undercover in Vista taking the photos, which he sent to me to forward to Miguel in Ensenada, but not before I examined every single shot myself, first. It was astonishing to me how much Sylvia resembled the woman in the composite sketch. *Miguel might be right about her,* I thought.

My sisters were feeling the same sense of urgency and frustration that I was. I emailed them as soon as I got off the phone to share my outrage about Detective Long and my gratefulness for Eduardo Reyes. It was getting more and more difficult for my sisters and me to remain optimistic and upbeat, but we made it a practice to see and talk with one another often and plan for fun occasions. We were acutely aware that a tragedy like the one we were all living through could easily tear a family apart, and we were determined not to let that happen to us.

In fact, we were closer than we had ever been. Debbie and Sherri's birthdays were both in July and were opportunities for us all to gather. Mom always said that Sherri was the smartest of us girls, with the highest IQ, and Sherri's intelligence was matched by her quick wit and cleverness. Sher decided that her birthday this year would surround a theme—a "Sher"-lock Holmes theme. Sherri's married name is Holmes, so it was perfect. We enjoyed our time together, but as happened on every occasion for celebration in 2006, my sisters and I spent the majority of the "party" talking and strategizing about our next move in Mom's case. I recounted the story that Eduardo had told me about his trip to San Felipe and outlined my desire to help our Mexican detectives in any way possible, surmising if SDSO was not going to investigate, then we might just have to do it ourselves. That night, Deb, Sher, Kim, and I began to talk seriously about taking a trip to Puertecitos to see where Mom died.

I had taken Eduardo's words about Ortiz, Velez, and Espinoza to heart, and by the end of summer began to have regular correspondence and calls with Miguel Ortiz. On one call Miguel told me Velez and Espinoza had used the photos of Sylvia Murphy to perform photo line-ups and re-interview witnesses in San Felipe. The detectives had placed six photos, including one of Sylvia, in front of witnesses for review, and they were asked to pick out one that resembled the person of interest.

At the Hotel Costa Azul, where Mom was reported to have stayed, the desk clerk who claimed that she checked Mom and the heavy set woman into the hotel, picked Sylvia out of the line up without hesitation. Miguel encouraged me to continue to put pressure on SDSO and the FBI, writing letters and making calls to ask for assistance in the case because it helped to keep focus. I assured Miguel that everything possible was being done from my end, and that in fact my husband had just forwarded a letter to a family friend in government, a former Governor and White House Chief of Staff, who would be meeting in the coming week with the San Diego area Congressman in Washington, DC, to discuss the lack of movement on Mom's case on behalf of our family.

My indignance over Burt Long's cavalier attitude about Mom's case began to consume me, and I decided to reach out in all directions. I had asked for Rick's help in contacting Congressman Darrell Issa because I hoped that we could get the FBI's assistance on the case. Like many Americans, I assumed if something happened to a US citizen in a foreign country the FBI would be there to assist local authorities. Saddened by the disappearance of

Natalee Holloway and curious about the FBI's role in the investigation, I picked up the book, *Aruba: The Tragic Untold Story of Natalee Holloway*, co-authored by Dave Holloway and Larry Garrison, and read it quickly cover to cover. One afternoon, while the kids were out with friends at the beach, I decided to pick up the phone and call Mr. Garrison myself and ask him about how the FBI had come to investigate in Aruba.

I was surprised at how quickly a computer search gave me his number. I dialed and he answered the line himself.

"Larry Garrison," he said.

"Hello, Mr. Garrison, my name is Lauri Taylor. Do you have a moment?"

"What is your call in regard to Ms. Taylor?"

"My mother was murdered in Mexico six months ago, and I wondered if I could ask you a few questions."

"I'm so sorry to hear about your mom. Tell me how I can help you."

I poured out Mom's story to him as quickly as I could, not sure how long his generosity would last. He asked me many questions about the case and shared stories of families he had worked with in the past. After about an hour, I finally rounded back to the question I really wanted answered.

"How did the FBI become involved in Aruba?" I asked.

"The Aruban government invited the FBI to assist in the investigation. A request must come from the country where the crime occurs. The FBI cannot simply step into another country to investigate."

It was not the answer I had hoped to hear, but I thanked Mr. Garrison for his time and advice, and he kindly asked that I keep him abreast of any developments in the case.

The call with Mr. Garrison left me feeling as though my sisters and I could add the FBI to the growing list of law enforcement agencies that would not be helping us anytime soon. If we were going to find answers, most assuredly we would have to find some of them ourselves. I arranged a conference call with my sisters and Chris Mendoza in August to discuss plans for a trip to San Felipe and Puertecitos. We agreed that it was time to take matters into our own hands and marked our calendars for a girls' road trip to Mexico for the middle of September.

ELEVEN

Girls' Trip to Mexico

Our girls' road trip to Mexico began in typical girl fashion—at least it was typical for the girls in our family: we were all running late. Chris patiently waited as we loaded our overnight bags into the back of my SUV along with Sherri's signature snacks and refreshments from Trader Joe's. It was Sher's position that we could not be "Super Sleuths" if we had low blood sugar; our brains just simply wouldn't function as well. Debbie arrived for our girls' trip with an equally bright outlook, wearing a "CSI" investigator ball cap and carrying a note pad. She was ready to investigate, which made us all laugh. Kim was her usual funny self, doing impressions in a combination of Spanish and English, with lots of mentions of tequila. We were all doing what we had been trained to do—we were putting a great face on a difficult situation, making it look easy. My sisters and I were going on a hunt for clues about our mother's murder, but to anyone who may have witnessed us loading up the car that day, we simply appeared to be a group of women (and one ex-Marine in another vehicle) headed south for a "fun" weekend in Mexico.

And we did have fun. Cruising down the highway toward the border, we reminisced about our lives with Mom and about the shock of finding ourselves in the middle of a murder investigation. We stopped for gas just before the border to fill up and bought "mood" rings to wear on our adventure, and when we got back on the road, Kimi promptly revealed she was in a black mood, which made us bust up, again. One point that struck me as funny while listening to my sisters chat our way down the highway was that we had all learned as much from our mother when she was *not* there for us as we had when she was actually there for us. We had become strong, resilient, and resourceful because we were forced to be. *Mom would be proud of us*, I thought, *for not accepting Burt Long's indifference about her case, and taking the reigns of the investigation into our own hands.*

We checked into the Hacienda Don Jesus in the afternoon on Friday. Deb and I gave Kim and Sherri the tour of what had been our home away from home for the time we had spent there in March. Chris, my sisters, and I had already decided that our trip to Puertecitos would begin Saturday morning, and so we headed to the Malecon to eat and poke around a bit. Passing by the Ministerio Público on our walk brought back a lot of memories for Deb and me that we shared with Chris, Sher, and Kim, laughing about the ridiculousness of meeting Octavio and our ride to the morgue. Deb and I intended to share all of the places and memories from our crazy three days in San Felipe with Sher and Kim, and to interview as many people as we could who might remember something about our mother's stay there, as well.

I realized very quickly that we had made a huge mistake by not bringing a translator on the trip with us; we needed to have very precise conversations, and with me translating that would not be possible. This could not have been more evident than when we arrived at the Hotel Costa Azul to speak with a witness. Debbie and I had walked right past it when we walked on the Malecon in March, but at the time, we had no idea that this was the hotel where the investigators suspected Mom had stayed. Deb, Sher, Kim, Chris, and I walked into the lobby of the hotel hoping to speak with the clerk who we were told had checked Mom in, and hoping to find anyone else who might remember seeing Mom. I approached the front desk and told the woman behind the counter that we would like to speak with the clerk who had helped our mother. I explained in my best Spanish that she had been killed (or I might have said she had mutated—the verbs are a lot alike in Spanish) near Puertecitos, but the woman actually understood right away with whom I wanted to speak.

"Queria hablar con Esmeralda," she said. *You want to speak with Esmeralda.*

"O, si." *Oh yes,* I said. "Cuando trabaja ella, siguiente?" *When does she work next?*

"Ella trabaja hoy, a las cuatro de la tarde," she said. We had gotten unbelievably lucky. Esmeralda, the clerk responsible for giving the description of the person of interest to the artist who drew the composite picture for Mexican authorities, would be working her shift later that day.

My sisters and I decided to make good use of our time while we waited to speak to Esmeralda, and so we headed straight out to shop and grab a beer. We strolled in and out of the little trinket shops along the boardwalk. Kim and I bought matching camouflage jammies, a family tradition for special occasions and holidays. Kim bought her favorite pink camo and I bought the blue camo because we felt like we were going to battle for our mom. We sat in the café bar where Debbie and I had sat when we got the call from Ben Cook about Karla Nelson's photos. We ordered lunch and our beers and discussed our priorities for the remainder of the weekend. After lunch, we took a walk to point out Octavio's

farmacia on our way back to the Hotel Costa Azul for our interview of Esmeralda.

Esmeralda was a pretty young girl with milky brown skin, long
coarse brown hair, and disarming emerald green eyes. She smiled at
me when I approached the desk, and it was obvious she knew who
we were and was not intimidated at all by our presence.

"Mucho gusto, soy Lauri," I said. *Pleased to meet you, I'm Lauri.*

"Mucho gusto, soy Esmeralda," she said, smiling again, and
although this is where the ease of our exchange ended, we managed to piece it together.

I asked Esmeralda if she could tell us about seeing our mom. My
sisters and I had heard Miguel Ortiz's description of Esmeralda's
explanation of the day—she said Mom checked into the Hotel
Costa Azul—but we needed to hear it directly from her.

Esmeralda pointed in the direction of the covered driveway
and began to describe what she had seen, not only with her words,
but using her hands to show us what she meant, as well.

"Your mom pulled in and parked the green car at the curb. She
came to the desk and asked for a room for the night. She wanted
a view of the water and pulled out her credit card to pay. Just then
a big woman, who had gotten out of the passenger side of the car,
came to the desk and said, "No, no, let me pay for that," and gave
me cash for the room. The woman with your mom was wearing
short pants, a plaid shirt and baseball hat. Your mom stepped away
from the desk, and walked to the couch over there and sat down,"
Emeralda said, pointing to a seating area in the lobby.

"Your mom pulled her glasses from the top of her head and
wrote in a small notebook while she sat there waiting."

I stood there stunned by Esmeralda's description of my mother's exact physical mannerisms. I had goose bumps. Deb, Sher,
Kim, and I exchanged looks of disbelief, but it was not disbelief

about what she said that we were feeling. We were amazed at how perfectly she had captured something we could all so easily imagine our mom doing. How could she have known Mom had a tiny notebook? I had seen it in Mom's purse when Deb and I were sitting in Jorge Silva's office. In that moment we were all convinced that our mother had spoken to this young woman and had stayed at the Hotel Costa Azul. *Esmeralda could not possibly have been coached by anyone to convey what she had just shown us. If she was right about that, how could she not be right about the woman with whom Mom was traveling, as well? Was Sylvia Murphy here with Mom?*

Esmeralda continued and explained that a security guard followed Mom and the other woman out as they parked their car in the courtyard. He said that when the hatch of the van was opened, there were brown suitcases and shopping bags in the back. The same security guard had seen the two women in the parking lot, later during their stay, having an argument. One calling the other a "bitch." At some point, the heavyset woman had come back to the reception desk and paid cash for an additional night when Esmeralda was not working. No one recalled seeing the women check out of the hotel, and there was no record of their stay because they paid cash.

I wondered if she remembered what Mom had been wearing, so I asked her to describe it. Esmerelda told me that Mom was wearing a cream colored camisa, which we found surprising. Mom had been photographed at the ATM in Vista on March 14, wearing her bright red sweat outfit, the same one her body was found in on March 24, but that was not what Esmeralda had described.

"Muchas gracias por su ayuda," I said, thanking her for her help.

"De nada, su madre era muy hermosa," she said. *You're welcome, your mother was very beautiful.*

I turned to Deb, Kim, and Sher, choked up. "She said Mom was very beautiful," I said, and we all left the hotel in tears.

Saturday morning, we loaded up and headed south out of town towards Puertecitos. Chris led the way in his truck. As we passed by little hotels on the outskirts of San Felipe, I wondered to myself if any of them were the place where Eduardo had stayed with his motorcycle-riding buddies. We discussed the possibility of Mom coming to San Felipe to buy real estate as we whipped past the numerous "for sale" signs along the highway. Not far down the road, though, the landscape became quite desolate and I was again extremely thankful that Mom's body had been found at all. The pastor's explanation for staying with Mom's body because of the packs of coyotes that roam the area at night now seemed completely plausible.

The Sierra San Pedro Martir mountain range, the western boundary of the San Felipe Desert, hugged the coast on our right and the beautiful blue green water of the Sea of Cortez was to the left as we rolled down the highway. The further South we drove, the worse the surface of the road became, and it narrowed to practically a single lane for two cars to pass on. The potholes grew larger by the mile, increasing to the size of craters that threatened to swallow up my car. I gripped the steering wheel tighter and slowed my car to a snail's pace, secretly wishing that I were simply a passenger, not the driver and translator.

Come to think of it, my sisters were probably no more comfortable riding as passengers on that road than I was. Debbie and Sherri wrote notes everywhere we went, writing down our questions and observations, but it was becoming more difficult to ignore where we were headed even as we tried to keep the mood light.

One after another, we passed the campos that were lined up along the beachfront of the Sea of Cortez. Most of the campos were simply a plot of land to pitch a tent on or pull up a trailer, but a handful of them had "permanent" home-like structures. Each was marked with a unique sign to distinguish one campo from another, some clever and well made, others, simple and nondescript. Instead of addresses the campos had names, and property lines were differentiated by kilometer markers. Mom's body had been found in Campo Zimmaron, at KM marker 68, not in the city of Puertecitos as we had originally been told by the district attorney of San Felipe. We had wrongly imagined her in an actual city, not the wide-open expanse of desert wilderness we were in.

It turns out that "Puertecitos" was more of a ballpark generalization of the area, given for the sake of our family and US authorities who might be looking on a map. What became more evident to me as I drove was that it would be impossible for SDSO to speculate about possible scenarios without visiting the scene, and as far as I could tell, that was never going to happen.

I followed Chris down the long stretch of dirt road into Karla Nelson's campo and parked right next to Chris's truck. It had taken well over an hour to get to this point, and the girls and I were ready to get out of the car to stretch our legs and do some exploring. There were no other vehicles on the property, so we assumed that Karla and her husband were not home, but Chris went to the door to knock, just to confirm our suspicions. The single-story, mobile home type residence had a multicolored brick facade and sat only about fifty yards from the Sea of Cortez. My sisters spread out around the property, and I walked along the side of the building towards the beach where a small patio, with several windows and a door with iron grates, opened towards the beach. A stiff breeze off of the water blew in my face and made me shiver a bit, despite the fact that it was a warm fall day in Baja.

Just steps from the home in front of the patio, I came upon a huge, stark white whale skeleton stretched across the dark brown sand. Struck by the size of the bones, maybe twenty-plus feet long, and by the fact that they laid perfectly in a line, I imagined the poor animal must have beached itself and died right there in front of Ms. Nelson's home. The thought of the beautiful majestic animal breathing in its last breath right there was sobering. I didn't need a reminder of why we had come to Mexico, but the image of the bones lying in the sand left me hollow and shivering.

Bending down to pick up a sand dollar near my foot, I was amazed at how many perfect, whole shells covered the sand around it. I frantically scooped them up, gathering as many as I could hold, until I heard Debbie call my name.

"Come on Laur, let's go," she yelled from the other side of the building, and I ran clutching the shells carefully between my hands back to the car. *Katy will love these*, I thought, placing them carefully in the back of the SUV.

We knew from speaking with Miguel Ortiz that Karla Nelson's campo was adjacent to Campo Zimmaron, minutes away from the place where Mom died. The closer we got to kilometer marker 68, the more confused my sisters and I became about what would have brought Mom to this stretch of beautiful, but barren land. Just as our trip to the morgue had left Debbie and me with more questions than answers, this road trip was beginning to feel much the same.

The drive from San Felipe to this area of Baja was not a leisurely day trip that one would take alone. It was a brutal, scary drive in the daylight for four women in a sturdy SUV, but for a grandmother in a late-model minivan, it was unimaginable. *She had to be with someone,* I thought, *or following someone.* Just then, I saw Chris's blinker flash, indicating he was going to be turning left.

"There it is," Kim said at the exact same time, pointing to a white painted sign with a beautiful ram's head in the center and the word "Zimmaron" simply stenciled in the upper right-hand corner. A chill went up my spine. *This is the place.* I was struck by the irony of the ram—the spiritual sign of sacrifice and new beginnings. The only feeling this place evoked for me was a brutal, terrible ending. The eyes of the ram stared down on us as we drove past towards the water. Everything began to feel recognizable, the color of the vegetation and the sand and the rocks. I had looked at those thirteen photos only briefly and reluctantly, but I felt we were very close to the place where our mother had struggled and taken her last breath.

I pulled in closely behind Chris, worried about the depth of the sand where Mom's van had gotten stuck. I did not want to be stuck at Campo Zimmaron for a minute. My sisters and I sat chatting in the car before we opened our doors to get out. It made no sense to us that our mother had ended up in this place. One of the first questions that could be ruled out by our visit was that Mom had come for a leisurely camping trip, as detective Long had speculated. Although anchored on one side by the beautiful water of the Sea of Cortez, this place was desolate and fierce. Stepping out onto the dirt, my first thought was how thankful I was to have worn my Nikes. Sharp rocks and shells covered the brown dirt of the desert wash, the creek bed that was barren at that time of year. Mom would not have voluntarily walked barefoot here.

Chris had brought the thirteen crime scene photos to use as reference to locate the exact spot where Mom's body was found, and we all spread out in different directions to hunt the area for familiar landmarks. We tried to busy ourselves with the work of finding "the spot," but, from time to time Deb, Sher, Kim, and I were all overwhelmed with emotion, crying as we walked aimlessly, and at times, only pretending to search. We decided to go to Javier's Campo, which was the property just to the south of Campo Zimmaron, to see if we could find anyone home to ask about seeing Mom.

Although we could see the campo from the desert wash, we had to get back in our vehicles to drive there on the road because we feared getting stuck in the sand. Again, I trailed behind Chris's truck and watched him park in front of me near one of the structures on the property. Deb, Sher, Kim, and I burst out laughing when two dogs circled Chris's truck, lifted their legs, and peed on his tires.

"That just shows how they feel about us being here," Kim said, which left us all nearly hysterical with laughter when Chris walked back to my side of the car. I rolled down my window to speak with him, the dogs followed and christened my car as well, while we talked about what we would say when we got to the door.

After a brief introduction and conversation Javier and Lydia, his wife, volunteered to take us to the exact place where Mom's body was found. Javier (beer in hand), Lydia, and I jumped into his vehicle and he motioned for Chris to follow. Javier drove us back to almost the exact location we had been in minutes earlier, and when we got out of the car again, I knew we had arrived. I stood close to Lydia, a gentle, motherly woman with a rounded figure, probably acquired over years spent cooking for her family, and who had a sweet smile and calm demeanor. She began to speak to me softly in Spanish, watching Javier lead Chris and my sisters to a corner of the dry creek bed.

I leaned in to hear her better as she described how her son and daughter had been out in the morning hunting octopus, which was consistent with what we had been told by investigators. Her young daughter had run home, frightened by what she saw in the distance, a woman whose skin looked like porcelain, she said, touching her face for emphasis. Her little girl cried to her that she looked like a "muneca," a doll, lying there in the dirt in her bright red pants. My eyes filled with tears for Lydia's daughter, no older than Katy, who was disturbed by the image and still had "bad dreams."

"Lo siento," I sobbed, telling Lydia I was sorry. She reached out and hugged me while I cried.

"O Dios mio, no," she said, patting my back, reassuring me that it was not my fault, but I felt like it *was* my fault, and cried harder.

We walked together to where my sisters and Chris were huddled with Javier. Deb, Sher, Kim, and I hugged one another and cried. Javier asked us if we would like to leave something, a marker, where Mom's body had been found. We were not at all prepared for that question. It seemed too overwhelming a decision, and so we chose not to leave anything, but told Javier we would be back when we were more prepared. We hugged Javier and Lydia, thanked them for their help, and got back in our cars to get on the road to Puertecitos. But before we could even close the doors, Javier and Lydia invited us to come to their home. Surprised by their kind gesture, and hoping to ask them some direct questions, we accepted.

There were two structures on Javier's compound, each one a single story, grey brick building. Lydia welcomed us through the front door, and Chris, my sisters, and I filed in, single file. We entered into one large room that resembled a modest hunting cabin with a hodgepodge of mismatched furniture, collected trinkets from giveaways and travels, stickers, steins, and small statues. As Lydia welcomed us, Javier was turning over a large black mattress that had rested on top of the sofa, but when he started to flip the unwieldy frame, the black flew off the mattress, and a swarm of flies dispersed throughout the room. We all just kept smiling.

"Se sientan, por favor," Lydia said graciously—*Please take a seat*—inviting us to sit on the freshly uncovered sofa as Javier tossed the mattress into a corner of the room.

Javier and Lydia took seats in chairs that Javier pulled next to one another just across from the sofa, and suddenly I could feel the eyes on me. Everyone there was waiting for me to facilitate a conversation, to precisely ask and translate the questions we so needed answers to. But I was wiped out physically from the treacherous driving and emotionally from the time at the campo, and could barely muster a "Buenos Dias." The questions then began: *ask them this, ask them that, what did they say?*

I managed to translate a few things, but in every other sentence I stumbled, saying, "I'm sorry" in Spanish and English, apologizing in both directions for my inept facilitation of the conversation. The odd thing was that I totally understood nearly every word of Spanish spoken to me, but the words remained frozen in my brain while I chipped away word by word to offer the English version back to my sisters. Silently, I wished to be beamed up and out of that place to anywhere else in the world, but we were getting scraps of information, so I stuck with it.

Just as we were starting to make some progress in the conversation, another man entered the room. Javier and Lydia jumped up, respectfully, and introduced us to Luis, the local delegado, or deputy. Luis was dressed in light colored polyester slacks, the kind made popular by Jack Nicklaus back in the "day," and a collared shirt, his dark thin hair slicked back away from his face with some sort of shiny gel. Luis took the seat right next to Javier, leaning in over him. His physical presence instantly changed the mood in the room. Any time Javier would speak, Luis would interrupt him, laying his arm across Javier's body to stop him, and Lydia, who had offered very little from the start, became mute. *What was he afraid they were going to say?*

Just before Luis had entered the house, we were asking Javier about a man Debbie and I had encountered at the Ministerio Público back in March.

"Can you ask him about Julio?" Debbie said, in a whisper, turning her back to Luis.

Debbie and I met Julio in an office at the Minesterio Público when we were in San Felipe to identify Mom's body. Although small in stature, he was fit and imposing in his black t-shirt, with the words "Policia" printed in bright yellow stretched across his muscular chest. Julio had approached us in a kind manner to talk about Mom, but he had intimidated us both, telling Debbie and me that we should not go to Puertecitos because it was far too dangerous. Julio also told us that he had seen Mom when he was driving near Puertecitos on Wednesday, March 22, with his children who were riding in the back of his vehicle.

Through the rearview mirror, Julio claimed to have watched the kids wave to a woman, matching Mom's description, in a green van with the license plate RENES (Mom's license plate). Debbie and I became sentimental, easily picturing our mother, happy to see young children in the back of a car, smiling broadly and waving to them in her signature wave, not the typical back and forth across a chalkboard wave but one more like a puppet, nodding yes, up and down.

Julio had enthusiastically conveyed the story about seeing Mom in March, but later we discovered his recollection was completely inconsistent with the evidence and information we had accumulated in the past six months.

"Conoces a Julio?" I asked Luis. *Do you know Julio?*

"Si, le conozco," he said, confirming it.

Luis explained that Julio was young and mistaken about the dates. While he spoke he was leaning over Javier, who seemed to want to add something to the conversation, but stopped. Before Luis had entered, Javier told us that Julio was an aggressive cop. It made no sense to us why Julio would simply make up a story, but nothing quite made sense to us, and Julio's actions remained highly suspicious to me.

Luis had changed the tone in the room from warm hospitality to cool tolerance for our presence. The conversation became even more stilted and finally ground to a halt. My sisters and I exchanged glances during the awkward silence and took our cue to go. We thanked Javier and Lydia for their time, hugging them as we left.

I was the last one to get back to the car. Slumping into the driver's seat, exhausted, I pulled my door shut and realized that I had missed part of a conversation between my sisters.

"What do you think Javier meant by that?" Sherri said to Kim.

"Meant by what?" I asked, lost, looking over my shoulder into the back seat.

"When we were out on the wash earlier, while you were with Lydia, Javier told us, 'You know more than you think you know,'" Kim offered.

Just then Chris came to the window, which I rolled down again so we could speak to him.

"Are you ready to move on to Puertecitos?" he asked.

"Yes," we answered collectively.

"Javier is a good man," Chris said.

"What do you mean?" I asked.

"I offered him money to tell me anything he knew and he wouldn't take it."

"Wow, that is telling. We need to bring him something to thank him for his help today," Deb said.

"Let's pick up some beer in Puertecitos," Sher suggested.

We all agreed that beer was a good idea and jumped back on the dirt road to our destination.

Driving on to Puertecitos was a long and exhausting trip on a godforsaken highway. Just as we were rounding a turn, my eyes focused straight on the road ahead, Deb shouted, "Look at that sign! It says 'Octavio's Campo,'" and we all looked at once.

"What do you think the odds are that there is another man in this part of Baja with the name, Octavio?" she wondered a loud.

"You make an excellent point, Deb. Maybe our Deep Purple loving pharmacist/chauffeur knows more about the area and what happened to Mom, than he let on."

Approximately twenty minutes further into our drive, we spotted Puertecitos in the distance. Called, "The Little Port," it certainly looked as though it were going to live up to its name. Known for it's thermal, bubbling waters and boat ramp, Puertecitos was popular among fishermen and people who enjoyed motorcycles, sand rails, and watercraft. It was a modest little spot in the middle of nowhere, and my sisters and I had begun to get cranky by the time we arrived, possibly because we hadn't eaten in hours but more likely because we were so physically and emotionally spent.

We forced ourselves out of the car to take pictures surrounding the city sign and went to the local convenience store to buy beer for Javier. We also wanted to ask about the town and find out if anyone had information they could share with us about Mom. Our visit was not well received by the locals, and we learned very little from our stop there. We did learn the whereabouts of Cesar's home, the pastor who had stayed with Mom's body the night she was found, and jumped back in our cars to head that way. Driving out of town, one of us—possibly Sherri—nicknamed the unfriendly little town where we had been told our mother had died, "Puerte-fucking-citos," which we shortened to the acronym, "PFC" so as not to offend anyone from the area.

Chris and I spoke briefly with a petite woman at Cesar's house, conveniently located between Puertecitos and Javier's campo, where we were headed next to drop off the case of beer. She phoned Cesar by satellite to set up a time for us to meet him back at our hotel at 3:00. My sisters and I were very interested in getting the specific facts about when and how Mom's body had been discovered, and Cesar had not only been there, but he also spoke fairly decent English. Bingo! We jumped back in our cars and made our way to Javier's, and Debbie and Sherri went to the door to deliver his beer, which was a huge hit. Javier kindly invited them to stay, and they explained that we needed to get back to San Felipe for a meeting at 3:00.

We busted back as quickly as we could up the treacherous road and arrived just in time to meet with Cesar in our hotel restaurant. The pastor sat at the head of our long table, and we ordered drinks while he spoke, having to talk loudly because a mariachi band played in the far end of the room. Sherri sat across from me, taking notes on a large sketchpad. I was really losing focus and interest, as Cesar simply repeated information we had already heard from him about Mom. Cesar was telling us the story of marrying his wife when she was just thirteen years old, and we all cringed, barely able to conceal our collective disgust, when Sher tapped her Sharpie curtly on the pad in front of her to get my attention. I looked up, and she wrote the words, "My Way," on the paper, then said them out loud and poked her pen towards the band. My eyes filled to the brim and my body went slack, but I had to smile at the mariachi rendition of my mom's favorite Frank Sinatra song.

"And now, the end is here.
And so I face the final curtain.
My friend, I'll say it clear.
I'll state my case, of which I'm certain.
I've lived a life that's full.
I traveled each and every highway.
And more, much more than this, I did it my way."

And when I get back the States, I plan to do it my way, I thought.

TWELVE

꿍ꚩ

The Appeal

The emotional trip to Mexico had bonded my sisters and me even further. Without Mom in the middle, trying to draw alliances between her daughters by pitting us one or two against another, we were very much a team—dedicated to keeping all in the loop and respecting each other's opinions and input. But something bigger began to happen after Mexico: my sister's started to rely on me for the majority of the communications and decisions in Mom's case. Logic dictated that I would be the one to take the position of case manager, because I lived closest to San Diego and Mexico, I spoke Spanish, and everyone assumed I had the time because "I didn't work." They were appreciative and encouraging, and I wanted to deliver a killer to my sisters as much as I wanted it for Mom and for myself.

I hit the ground running after returning from our trip to San Felipe, reenergized and suspicious as ever, of nearly everyone and their motives—every person in San Felipe, law enforcement on both sides of the border (save for Eduardo Reyes who would remain in a protected class of his own), all Mom's employees and acquaintances in Vista, and people I didn't even know. I spent my time after I dropped the kids at school firing off emails, searching the Internet, and making phone calls, but by mid-October frustration and doubt were at an all time high.

My sisters and I felt like we had three avenues of hope left in the investigation: America's Most Wanted, DNA results from San Diego Sheriff's Office, and the possible work with the California Department of Justice profiler. Many of my emails and calls went to Eduardo Reyes asking for his help and advice. As it became clear that Mom's case wasn't getting the attention we wanted from SDSO, I counted on his advice even more. He was a law enforcement insider who treated me with great respect and consistently honored my concern and frustration with the pace of the investigation. He reminded me quite often that it was my right to ask questions, and it was not too much to expect for people in law enforcement to do their jobs.

Although I was working hard on the case, my patience was wearing thin with SDSO, and on Friday, October 20th, I sent a terse email to the crime lab at SDSO requesting a call back regarding the DNA results. Four days later, I received a one-line response informing me that I should expect to receive a call back from the Homicide Unit. I called Chris right away and we agreed that we would both be on the call, so when Long called, I let it go to voicemail, and then Chris and I conferenced him back. And what a call it turned out to be.

"Detective Long."

"Hey, Burt. It's Lauri Taylor and I have Chris Mendoza on the line. How are you?"

We exchanged short pleasantries and got right to the point.

"Five bottles were tested in the lab and your mom's DNA was extracted from two bottles, but no other usable DNA was found."

"What does that mean?" I pleaded, knowing that the answer could not be good.

"We have done all we can do, and your mom's case is officially inactive."

My heart felt like it was on fire and I choked back my tears that had welled up because I dared not show Detective Long any weakness or vulnerability. *He does not know me, I do not give up that easily*, I thought.

"If it was your mother, what would you do?" I asked him directly.

"I would contact the FBI and the US Consulate."

"Do you have a number or a contact at the FBI?"

"No, I don't," he said.

★   ★   ★

As soon as Chris and I hung up with Long, I called Eduardo, completely distraught. He managed to talk me off the ledge and generously offered to send our crime scene photos to the DOJ profiler, which was really helpful because it was some sort of progress in the face of the big DNA dead end.

Another dead end that was particularly tough on Kim had to do with the television show, *America's Most Wanted*. She had been working for months—emailing, calling and using her work connections—to get *America's Most Wanted* interested in doing a story about Mom, but when the AMW producer, Michell Sigona, spoke with Burt Long, he told her that Mom's case was inactive and much to our collective disappointment, Ms. Sigona quickly lost interest in producing a piece.

Rick called me later that week to tell me he had received a message from Don McKinney at Congressman Issa's office and gave me the number to call back. While I was excited and thankful for Rick's help, I secretly feared we were headed for another dead end. How many dead ends would it take before we had to simply give up?

In early November, Don answered his direct line and we had a quick conversation about what my family was asking from the congressman's office.

"Lauri, I'm so sorry about your mother. How may I help you and your family?"

"Thank you and thank you to the congressman, as well. San Diego Sheriff's office has let my mother's case go inactive, essentially closing down their investigation, but we don't believe that everything has been done that can be done on this side of the border," I said.

"Let me speak with the undersheriff and I will get back with you," he said.

Don was good as his word and phoned back less than a week later with good news.

"I spoke with the undersheriff, Bill Gore, and you and your family will have the opportunity to appeal SDSO's decision to close the investigation," he said.

I was floored by the positive news. "When?"

"December 6, at SDSO headquarters. Can you email me a list of who will be attending with you?"

"Certainly, and thank you again for your help."

This appeal is something to be thankful for, I thought, something we desperately needed.

The family gathered at my house for Thanksgiving, as had become our tradition over the past several years. It was a holiday that Mom had particularly enjoyed and participated in. When we were growing up, Mom had always loved a house full of family, friends, and strays, as she called them, at every holiday.

Whoever did not have a place to spend Thanksgiving was always welcome at our celebration—a legacy I loved and tried to honor in my own home. The more the merrier was definitely our motto, too, and with a guest list of well over thirty, I would do my best to put out a great holiday dinner in a festive atmosphere, in her honor.

Despite our efforts, everything that day reminded my sisters and me of Mom, and we all walked around as though we were missing a limb, welling up with tears at every memory. Debbie made the pies that Mom had made every year since forever: apple and pumpkin, and sometimes, when she was in the mood, her beautiful lemon meringue, puffed high with fluffy egg whites and lightly browned on top. Who would make the rolls? I bought the frozen bread dough and had thawed it in the dry warm laundry room where it had puffed up and was ready to be hand rolled into Mom's signature dinner rolls. I could see her at my kitchen island with a dish towel draped over her left shoulder, elbow deep in flour, but still sipping from her glass of chardonnay and secretly dropping tiny bites of whatever she could grab to place in Bailey's mouth, even though I had asked her repeatedly not to give him treats.

With the dog at her feet wagging and Katy standing close by, Grandma Jane would show Katy, and whoever else was standing there chatting, how to pull the yeasty dough into small pieces, and with well floured hands, roll them into three perfect balls that she placed into the wells of the buttered muffin tin. Then she would place them back into the warm laundry room, and somehow they would rise again, triple in size, just in time to be baked while we cooked the green beans and mashed the potatoes, filling the house with the irresistible smell of fresh baked bread.

Oh my God, who is going to make the gravy? I thought. I had gathered the kids around to make the rolls and we had all cried over the bread dough, but then fell apart laughing at our lopsided, imperfect creations that Grandma Jane would never have allowed. The gravy was another matter, though. No one wanted the responsibility of making the gravy, but just as she had stepped up to make the pies, and as she had so many times in our life, Debbie stepped in to fill Mom's shoes on gravy, as well.

When Kim and I were freshmen in high school, Mom was going through a rough patch in her love life and in her work, which had crossed over a year earlier when Jane married one of her co-workers who was nearly ten years younger. Mom took their breakup hard, checking out of her motherly responsibilities, and Kim and I ended up in the care of our twenty-one-year-old sister, Debbie. It was a good six to nine months before Mom got her act back together and found a place for Kim and me to rejoin her, but Debbie just took it in stride, treating her little sisters to beef stroganoff dinners, sisterly advice, and lots of hugs. On Thanksgiving Day I was grateful to have the appeal to look forward to, but I was thankful for my sisters every day.

We got our Christmas tree on Sunday, December 3rd, because I anticipated that the week was going to be crazy busy with Katy's "Christmas Carol" rehearsals and performances, Clark's golf lessons, and Rick's annual trip to Tokyo for his work. While I was getting my haircut Wednesday morning, my stomach was in knots. Debbie, Sherri, and Kimi were swinging by my house that afternoon, and they had all mentioned that they would like for me to speak on behalf of the family. I was honored and proud that they would entrust me with the huge responsibility, but I was also scared to death and filled with self-doubt. A quick pep talk with Eduardo on Tuesday had helped me develop a strategy, but the bit of confidence I had picked up during our conversation had already dissipated. Eduardo warned me that he had seen families just like ours get the opportunity to appeal a case, then shoot themselves in the foot (the words of a sworn officer of the law) by being overly emotional and unprepared when it was their turn to present a rebuttal. I rushed home with my freshly flat-ironed hair, which always made me feel a bit more professional than my naturally frizzy locks, to write an outline.

Deb, Sher, and Kim came to pick me up about 1:00, and as we drove I gave them the review of Eduardo's caution about emotions. We all laughed and agreed that we were not above using emotion, though, if it was to our benefit. If things started to sway too far in Burt Long's favor, we all agreed that Kim would be the one who would sob on cue. She had us all in stitches doing her best dramatic imitation. I read through my outline from the passenger seat while Deb drove, and I told the girls that I had Googled Undersheriff Bill Gore over the weekend and discovered some information about him I thought might be helpful in our meeting.

The undersheriff had been the head of the San Diego field office of the FBI for many years prior to his position with SDSO, and his wife had been one of the first female FBI agents. Part of my strategy was to tell him that back in May, I had consulted the opinion of former FBI profiler, Gregg McCrary, who had examined the thirteen Karla Nelson photos and had spoken briefly about Mom's case with Detective Long. Mr. McCrary was deeply involved in the case of George Smith, a honeymooner who had mysteriously disappeared from a cruise ship, but had given me his opinion about the crime scene. He told me that he believed our suspect to be an acquaintance (versus a stranger) and therefore we had a finite suspect pool and a highly solvable crime. I felt strongly that the allegiance among FBI agents ran deep, and hoped the opinion of a fellow agent would convince the undersheriff to take another look at Mom's case.

The drive went by far too quickly, as time always does when we are anticipating something we dread, like a visit to the dentist's office. Sweet Eduardo, dressed in his plaid button down and slacks, met us in front of the San Diego Sheriff's office headquarters and escorted us to the front desk lobby to collect our badges. It was comforting to have him there for moral support because he believed as we did that Mom's case had not been fully investigated by SDSO. There were several people mingling about in the lobby, and as soon as we had signed in to receive our credentials, a tall, dark-haired man in a suit approached our group.

"Hello, are you Mrs. Kling's family?" he said to all of us.

"Yes, we are," Deb said.

"I'm Don McKinney, from Congressman Issa's office," he said with a smile.

"Hello, Don," I said, extending my hand, "I'm Lauri Taylor. Thank you so much for being here for us." I introduced him to my sisters and Eduardo.

"I'm happy to be here," he said.

Just as we began to chat with Don, an SDSO officer greeted our group, escorted us onto the elevator, and informed us that the undersheriff would be available to meet with us in just a few minutes. We were all asked to wait in a small reception area just off of the elevator. I had hoped to have the opportunity to ask Don about what to expect from our meeting with the undersheriff, but I could hardly breathe, I was so nervous, and so I made small talk instead. *How the hell am I going to speak?* I thought. Almost precisely at 3:00, Undersheriff Bill Gore stepped off the same elevator we had just left. He was an imposing figure, broad chested and very tall, probably 6´ 3˝ or so, or maybe he just seemed larger because I was feeling intimidated. He had soft blue eyes and a wide smile.

"Hello, I'm Bill Gore," he said, reaching to shake each of our hands warmly. "And this is Lt. Ethan D'Agostino," he added, introducing the dark eyed, very Italian, balding gentleman over his shoulder.

"I believe you all have met in the homicide division conference room before but today, we will be in the larger conference room down the hall."

Following closely behind him, I clutched a small file folder with my hastily typed outline inside, and wished I were any place any place but the San Diego Sheriff's Office. *Why do we need a large conference room for our little group?* I wondered, but understood very quickly as soon as we stepped in through the double doors and were directed to take our seats. The room was packed with people, but only on one side. A huge projection screen hung from the ceiling in the center of the room, perfectly dividing the horseshoe-shaped conference table into halves—ours and theirs.

A picture of my mom's beaten, strangled, half-clothed body, laying in the rocky soil of a dessert wash, shone on the canvas. "Welcome to the Homicide Division, Girls," it screamed at me. *Was this necessary? What was the point? Were they trying to intimidate us?* On their side, seemingly every member of the unit, mostly men, were crowded two rows deep in their seats, trying to get a look at us. We sat directly across from Burt Long, who looked smug—he always looked smug—tucked comfortably in amongst his colleagues. Even the three investigators from Ensenada were seated on the other side of the room. They smiled and waved. Eduardo walked in the door and took his seat in the corner of the room on our side, just behind Don McKinney, and I felt a slight bit of relief.

Quick introductions were made, and we were told that the homicide division would give a quick overview of the case; then our family would have an opportunity to present our appeal. Jim Hargreaves, from SDSO, started right in with his summation of the facts and Deb, Sher, Kim, and I looked at one another, trying to remain respectful, but trading subtle glances of disbelief, as he spoke. The problem was that the officer had most of the basic facts and dates wrong, like what day Mom had been reported missing and when her vehicle had crossed into Mexico. When Hargreaves concluded, he was just about to hand off to Burt Long, when Debbie cautiously raised her hand to speak.

"Would you like for us to correct the discrepancies in facts and dates now, or do you prefer for us to wait until it is our turn to speak?" she asked sincerely.

"You will have the opportunity to clarify later," the undersheriff said.

Detective Long smiled weakly at Debbie and began to speak, directing most of his commentary towards the undersheriff and Don McKinney, and occasionally looking across to our side of the room. The picture that Burt painted was that our mom had voluntarily gone to San Felipe, possibly in an altered state from the Soma, and was the victim of a random act of violence or a crime of opportunity, commenting that Mom had a nice little hooch that she stayed under, as if she was out in the wilderness camping. Not once did detective Long refer to the huge screen that hung in the room, and I wondered again why that awful picture had to be shining there above us.

When Detective Long had finished, Deb, Sher, Kim, and I asked some questions, and Deb did indeed have a chance to clarify the errors that had been made earlier. Then all eyes were suddenly on me; it was my turn to rebut Detective Long as he sat there among his fellow officers. I gathered my thoughts for a moment and remembered Eduardo's advice—no emotion, just the facts. I began to speak, my knees and voice quivering from the full weight of Mom's case heaped upon my shoulders, and took a deep breath in.

"First of all, I would like to thank everyone for being here today. My family and I truly appreciate your work on our mother's case and we fully understand the limitations we face: two countries, two languages, and at least two law enforcement agencies and all the jurisdictional questions that come with them, but we would like to formulate a plan to move forward with the investigation."

I canvassed the room as I spoke. My gaze was met and challenged with the icy glares of cops who, I imagined, were not happy to have their work scrutinized by an Orange County housewife. I immediately noticed a man sitting in the second row, directly behind Detective Burt Long, and I assumed his choice of seats, right next to his colleague's, indicated he was there to support Detective Long, but could not figure out who he was. Leaning back, legs casually crossed, he hadn't been introduced at the beginning of the meeting with the other top brass from Homicide. Not your typical sheriff's office veteran, thick in the middle from too many hastily grabbed fast-food lunches, he was fit and tan, conservatively dressed in a pale-blue, oxford cloth button-down shirt, neatly pressed but not stiff with starch like a Wall Street executive; he seemed relaxed and open. He gently smiled and nodded, his vibrant blue eyes softened, and I felt bolstered by his compassionate expression. I steadied myself and continued, but wondered, "*Who is this guy and why does he appear to actually be interested in what I have to say?*"

"As it stands now, the two law enforcement agencies are working on mutually exclusive theories. The SDSO theory you have heard today from Detective Long. The theory from Ensenada is that our mother had no connections or ties to Mexico, and the last person she was seen with in San Felipe was an American. We have had a composite sketch and a person of interest since our meeting in April, who has not been re-interviewed since our mother's body was found. My family would simply like to rule her out as a suspect or gather enough evidence to call her a legitimate suspect."

The stranger continued to listen intently, fully engaged, looking me in the eye, as I outlined each point about the department's handling of Mom's case, and somehow I knew his interest was genuine. A completely unfamiliar yet friendly face, in a room full of now vaguely familiar but unfriendly faces, put me at ease, and I pushed on.

"Two separate, highly regarded profilers, retired FBI agent Gregg McCrary and the profiler for the California Department of Justice, have looked at our crime scene photos and told us we have a highly solvable crime, a finite suspect pool, and that a crime of opportunity was unlikely," I said, now looking directly at the undersheriff for emphasis.

Bill Gore appeared to sit up a bit in his seat, and I wrapped up my thoughts.

"We don't believe that our mom's case has been fully investigated, as we have been asking for help since April to acquire the landline phone records, the surveillance video from the grocery store, additional DNA processing, and we have asked for the questioning of Mom's friend's and associates. Thank you all for your time."

The undersheriff pushed back his chair and stood up to conclude the meeting. "There is obviously still work to be done on your mother's case," he said, "and your family will have the full support and cooperation of the San Diego Sheriff's Department."

When the undersheriff had finished speaking, the meeting broke up. The stranger stood and strode casually over in his khaki slacks with his arm outstretched to shake my hand. "Hello, I'm Ray Henry, the sergeant in charge of Homicide," he said. Relieved and overjoyed by the news from the undersheriff, I fully hugged him, as did, Debbie, Sherri, and Kimi. We were giddy, and Deb told Ray, "Sorry, we're a bunch of huggers," and we all laughed. I had a quick chat with him before we left the conference room, and Ray encouraged me to call him anytime about the case. And I believed he meant it.

Eduardo wanted to have a quick chat with the DA and the detectives from Mexico, whom we also hugged, before he left.

Eduardo asked us to wait and meet him out in front of the building. When he walked up a few minutes later, he had a big proud grin on his face as if his protégés had just won the blue ribbon.

"I have never seen anything like that before," he said. You all so graciously put them to shame. I loved it when you raised your hand," he said, looking at Debbie with a wink. "And you nailed it perfectly," he said, smiling at me. I thought I would burst with pride.

My sisters had trusted me to coordinate all the principals at the appeal meeting, and more importantly, they had asked me to be the voice of the family. This was an entirely new dynamic for me, the baby, whose opinion seemed to be rarely if ever asked for when we were growing up. I felt a great sense of responsibility to keep the ball moving on Mom's case. I found my voice and my purpose in that conference room. *And best of all,* I thought, *I had done it my way.*

Thursday, December 7, Kim sent me the greatest email:

"You were en fuego yesterday. Bringing the meeting together is one major thing, but the way you delivered our message was what brought it home. You go girl, and thanks for letting us put you in the 'hot' seat!"

In the late afternoon on Christmas Eve, Rick drove, and I sat in the passenger seat for the one hour drive up the 405 freeway to Sherri and Keith's house. Katy and Clark were begging from the backseat for Rick to turn on their favorite radio station while I sat thinking about the busy month, exhausted but pleased by all that had been accomplished—the meeting at SDSO, the follow-up correspondence and calls, Christmas prep and shopping for my kids so they could have a happy holiday with all the trimmings.

Staring out the window, daydreaming, I caught a glimpse of a woman's profile in the car next to us as it passed by, and my heart began to race. The woman was the spitting image of my mother— short cropped hair and freckled but slightly tanned skin—and for a brief second, I believed it was her. I carefully sat up in my seat to get a second look, hoping Rick and the kids wouldn't notice what I was looking at, embarrassed that I was seeing things, but the car was too far ahead. Tears spilled down my face as it got farther and farther out of sight.

I won't give up, I thought. *I won't.*

THIRTEEN

~⟨⟩~

The Experts

Nine months had gone by since Mom's murder. Our family rang in the New Year of 2007, and while we were no closer to an answer about our mother's murder, it finally felt as though we were gaining a little momentum. The victory of re-opening Mom's case had given the family a much needed morale boost, along with the added bonus of a new ally at SDSO, Sergeant Ray Henry. My sisters and I continued to diligently follow up with law enforcement and the news media on every development of the investigation.

Late in December 2006 one of Debbie's clients, Dave, suggested that she speak about Mom's case with his tennis buddy, Pete Noyes, an investigative reporter at Fox News. Pete was very interested in Mom's case, and after speaking with Debbie he offered to produce an investigative special to be aired prior to the one-year anniversary of Mom's death. Debbie then referred Pete to me for a more detailed breakdown of the facts of the case. We set up a time to talk.

I wanted to know all there was to know about Pete Noyes, and as had become my practice prior to any meeting or call, I sat down at my laptop and Googled him. There was a mountain of information available and my screen filled with his amazing credentials, awards, stories, and scoops that Pete had garnered over his thirty-plus year career. He had won multiple Emmys, a Peabody Award, the Edward R. Murrow award for his work about the Manson murders, and was a *New York Times* best-selling author of a book about the Kennedy Assassination, *Legacy of Doubt: Did the Mafia Kill JFK?* One of the most fascinating bits of information I gathered was that Pete had been the inspiration for the character Lou Grant, the gruff news director played by Ed Asner on *The Mary Tyler Moor Show.*

Our first real conversation was an incredible mix of questions, stories, and validation from a kind gentleman journalist who behaved much more like a caring father figure than a grumpy news hack like Lou Grant. I summarized all the details of the investigation for Pete, who was complimentary about my recollection of the facts and the thoroughness of my presentation, especially given that I was discussing my own mother. Pete's kindness and enthusiasm for Mom's story, as well as his clear desire to help any way he could with the investigation, put me at ease.

"I'm really afraid that we will never know what happened to Mom," I said, swallowing my tears, not wanting to appear unprofessional.

"You stick to it, Lauri, and you will have your answers," he said gently, breaking into a story about a cold case he had worked that had been solved more than fifteen years later.

I'm not sure I can wait that long, I thought.

Pete Noyes had worked closely with some of the best detectives in the law enforcement community, and I quickly gathered from him that murder is a business. And like any other business, there are professionals and experts, and there are scammers. Pete generously offered to make personal introductions to his distinguished colleagues in the murder business, because he wanted me to have the benefit of the best opinions and advice about moving forward in Mom's case. I was honored and entirely intimidated when Pete suggested I speak with his dear friend Leroy Orozco.

"Leroy is a former LAPD detective, and has worked some of the city's most infamous murder investigations," Pete said, "He was a member of the elite Night Stalker task force, and was present at the arrest and interview of Richard Ramirez, one of the most prolific serial killers in history."

Pete was proud of his friend's long list of accomplishments and successes in law enforcement, but as he casually outlined the accolades, all I could think was, *Why does Pete believe I am qualified to talk with this man about anything?*

"On the day Ramirez was taken into custody," Pete continued, "Leroy called me directly, and I was one of the first journalists on the scene to cover the breaking news story of the Night Stalker's capture and arrest."

"That is amazing, Pete. What a story."

"He has been in this business a long time, Lauri, and he will be able to advise you about using the composite sketch in our news piece."

"Okay, Pete, thank you. I will call Leroy in the morning after I get my kids off to school."

Pete was adamant about his desire to put the composite sketch on television, but the drawing had not been made public in the United States, and to complicate matters further, Ray Henry was not wholly in favor of using the composite because he didn't fully trust how it had been acquired from San Felipe and wanted witnesses to come forward without the bias of the sketch. I was trying to build a working relationship with Ray, and was worried that going against him on this decision might jeopardize his enthusiasm for helping us with Mom's case.

My sisters weren't convinced that using the composite sketch was the best strategy, either, but for different reasons than Ray Henry's. Our trip to Mexico had left my sisters and me pretty convinced that the woman in the composite was indeed Sylvia Murphy, and we were fearful that showing the sketch on television might tip Sylvia off and cause her to flee. We desperately needed another professional opinion, and despite my trepidation about speaking to the veteran homicide detective, I dialed Leroy.

Much to my surprise and relief, Leroy was a sweet, soft-spoken gentleman whose compassion for our plight was apparent from the moment he picked up the line. He had been briefed by Pete and patiently asked me to fill in some important elements of the investigation. Leroy was complimentary of Mexican sketch artists, naming a few in particular, and felt strongly that it was time to use the composite on air since no witnesses had come forward in almost a year. He recommended that we frame the piece as though we didn't have any inclination whatsoever who the person was in the sketch. Leroy thoughtfully told me to call him with questions any time and referred me to another retired detective named Charlie Sosa whom he had worked with and was a native Spanish speaker with contacts in Mexico.

My sisters and I agreed to allow Pete to release the composite on air, and I coordinated the logistics of the shoot with Miguel Ortiz, receiving permission for Pete's news anchor, Gina Silva, to interview District Attorney Morales and Detective Velez. Having learned from our girls' trip to San Felipe that I was not comfortable with the full responsibility of translating conversations, and because Deb, Sher, and I were worried about three women driving to Ensenada alone, I hired Burt Sosa to accompany us and to serve as our interpreter for the day of the shoot. Kimi, who worked for one of the top PR firms in Los Angeles representing celebrity clientele, had several big projects in the works, and was disappointed she could not take the time away to be there with us. We always felt better when the four sisters were together, and were proud of the fact that we were still there for one another. Burt met us at my house, and I was thrilled when he offered to drive.

Miguel Ortiz had assured me that his office was ready for Pete and his news crew, but I was anxious to get to the PGJE because history had shown that situations are entirely subject to change without notice in Mexico. After the two hour and fifty-five minute drive, we pulled up next to the Fox 11 News van, which was parked on the street in front of the offices of the PGJE. I recognized Pete right away from the photos I had seen of him on the Internet, but he was much shorter than I had imagined the man with the booming voice to be. I was grateful that he was already busy at work directing his crew when we walked up to introduce ourselves.

"Hello," he said, surveying the group, "Which one of you is Debbie?"

"I'm Debbie," she said, reaching out to shake Pete's hand.

"Dave has some very nice things to say about you," he said, shaking her hand and referring to his tennis partner and Deb's client.

"Which one of you two is Lauri?" he asked, looking back and forth between Sherri and me.

"I'm Lauri," I said, smiling and shaking his hand, "Nice to finally meet you, Pete."

"It's very nice to meet you, too. You have done a great job pulling this together young lady. We are just about set up and ready to shoot."

"Thank you, I'm happy it all came together," I said.

"Then, you must be Sherri," Pete said.

"We can't thank you enough for doing this for our family," she said.

Pete smiled. "It's the least I can do for you girls."

Alejandro Morales and Miguel Ortiz were both interviewed for the show, and Charlie did an excellent job of translating, making sure Deb, Sher, and I were aware of what was being said at all times. Pete insisted on getting on-camera interviews with Jane's daughters, which was always a bit unnerving, no matter how many times I stepped in front of a television camera. He also wanted a shot of the girls inside the office of the PGJE looking at evidence in the case. I don't know how Pete did it, but Morales pulled Mom's purse from their evidence locker and allowed us to rifle through the contents while being filmed. As canned as it may have seemed, Deb, Sher, and I all balled our eyes out when we saw the purse; Mom's wallet and the envelopes that had been found near Mom's body, and it was all caught on tape. Morales allowed my sisters and me to take the purse home with us and returned the money that had been found in Mom's socks. After Pete shot all the footage he needed, Charlie, Deb, Sher, and I took our detectives out for a steak lunch in Ensenada. Velez and Espinoza appreciated our gesture and were quite animated when discussing details of their investigation with Charlie.

Traveling to Ensenada with Charlie Sosa to do the Fox news story earned me greater credibility with Miguel Ortiz, Alejandro Morales, and Detectives Velez and Espinoza. Charlie was a veteran detective from the United States who spoke to them comfortably and respectfully in their own language. Just a week after we had returned from Ensenada, Morales offered to give the family a copy of the border-crossing video, which showed Mom's van at the border at Calexico/Mexicali, in hopes that we would have it professionally enhanced. Investigators believed it showed our mom and two other individuals get out of the van at the border crossing. I was astonished that the lead investigator would hand such valuable evidence directly over to me, but I had begun to expect unusual occurrences.

Charlie Sosa and I drove back to Ensenada to pick up the tape, and during the trip I overheard part of a phone conversation he had with an old friend who worked for the San Diego Police Department. He called the friend, Steve Lopez, and was asking if he had any contacts in San Felipe who might be able to help us. The name stuck in my brain, one of the many facts and bits of information I filed away in case it might someday do us some good.

One of the Taylor family's favorite perks of Rick's job was our annual trip to the Buick Invitational Golf Tournament at Torrey Pines. Rick, Clark, Katy, and I loved being in La Jolla for the tournament, walking the beautiful golf courses, eating our favorite "top secret" burger from the restaurant at the Lodge, and talking to the professional golfers in the hotel. That year it was a nice break away from the computer and the case for me, and a nice diversion while we waited for Pete's story to air in the next few weeks, but it also proved that try as I might, I really couldn't ever get away from those facts piling up in my mind. Standing next to the back entrance of the grandstand at the eighteenth hole, I waited with the crowd while ushers held up ropes to block the exit so players could move safely off of the green to the clubhouse. On either side of the path made by the ropes, policemen were stationed for security, and I found myself standing directly next to one of them. I smiled at the officer and glanced down at his nameplate: Steve Lopez. *It can't be the same guy,* I thought, *can it?* I was becoming bolder and decided to ask.

"Excuse me, you wouldn't happen to be friends with a retired officer named Charlie Sosa, would you?" I asked, as the ropes were lowered and the crowd made its way around me.

"Well, yes I am, as a matter of fact. And who might you be?"

"I'm Lauri Taylor, the client Charlie took to Ensenada last week," I said.

"Well, isn't it a small world," he said, "and I'm very sorry about your mother."

"Thank you, my family and I are doing what we can to find her killer."

He offered his encouragement, which was so kind, but I was still amazed that even on a weekend getaway, I couldn't get away from the case.

★   ★   ★

Pete's story was set to air on Saturday, February 10th, and in the weeks leading up to the airdate, Pete called me on a regular basis, asking for additional specifics about the people and facts surrounding Mom's disappearance to enrich his piece. He planned to take his news crew to Vista to get an official statement from SDSO, where he hoped to garner an on-camera interview with a top ranking official as well as footage of Mom's home and A&J Consignment. I gave Pete my contact information for SDSO and for Mom's landlord, Gene Rogers, because he wanted to have Gene's permission to film on his property.

I received a call from Pete after he had conducted interviews in Vista. "Lauri, it's Pete," he said, a bit breathless. "That guy Rogers went crazy on us. He held his hand over his waistband, pretending to have a gun, and threatened me and my cameraman."

"What, Pete? Why?"

"He said he was tired of people coming around his property."

"Wow, I'm sorry, Pete."

"Not to worry, Lauri, it's what I do, but I find his behavior highly suspicious."

"That is the problem Pete; it seems to us that everyone in Vista associated with Mom's case has acted suspiciously in one way or another. If we can't get San Diego Sheriff's Office to investigate in Vista, we can't rule out anyone as a suspect."

"I called SDSO about an official statement and left a message. No one ever called me back, but they did forward a statement from Lt. D'Agostino that was, to say the least, dismissive." Pete said.

"Can I trouble you to read it to me?" I asked.

"Of course, let me bring it up on my computer," he said and began reading, "We have cooperated with Mexican authorities (in the Jane Kling case), and we have processed some evidence for them. There is nothing new in the case. And there is nothing to suggest foul play occurred on this side of the border."

"How would he presume to know that no foul play occurred on this side of the border when his detectives haven't interviewed a single person since Mom's body was found?" I demanded.

"I can understand your frustration, Lauri. It just means you are going to have to keep pushing for answers."

I laughed. "You know I will, Pete," I said.

He paused and then said thoughtfully, "You're a real go-getter. You should have been a reporter."

I sucked in my breath, bolstered by his praise.

★   ★   ★

Sherri invited Deb, Kim, and me to gather at her house to watch Pete's news special with her husband Keith and Adam and Tiffany. I was happy to leave home since I did not want Clark and Katy to see the show. I feared the information would be overwhelming; it was too much for them to know about their grandmother. We were drinking wine, enjoying Sher's great food, and chatting about the investigation, when Keith turned on the television and the words "Anna Nicole Smith Found Dead in Florida" blazed across the wide screen. I was living partially in a bubble that revolved around my kids and the investigation, and I had not heard the news about Anna Nicole. It was heartbreaking to see the pictures of her beautiful baby, who would now be without a mother, but my thoughts went directly to a completely selfish place. *What a terrible night for Mom's news story to run—who will be watching?*

During a commercial break from reporting the latest news on Anna Nicole Smith, a promo ran for Mom's story and we all cheered, but ten minutes later, when Gina Silva spoke the words, "Murder Mystery in Mexico," we were silent as church mice, glued to the television screen. I personally think I held my breath for the entire thirty minutes. Pete had done exactly what he had promised us he would and framed the story as a complete mystery, as if we had no inclination of who the person of interest might be. Everyone seemed to be pleased with Pete's work and hopeful that the phone lines at Fox would be burning up with new leads by Monday. Everyone, that is, except Adam.

Adam sat back away from the group, and seemed even quieter than usual to me. I worried about Adam because I hadn't heard him speak much about Mom or the case, and I surmised that he was probably struggling with guilt about his relationship with his Grandmother as much as I was struggling with mine. Adam had been in the same place with Jane as I had been so many times in my life. He fluctuated between the idealized and prized grandson who, when strictly satisfying Mom's expectations, could do no wrong, and a much-maligned young man, when he was not. And I imagined that Adam wanted this nightmare over as much as I did, and that was good reason to get back to work.

★   ★   ★

March first came like a sledgehammer with the countdown to the one-year anniversary of Mom's death. Every morning over my first cup of coffee, I would run the times and facts of that particular date, one year earlier, through my head—where I was, where Mom was—and it was agonizing. I found myself looking at the clock throughout the day at the precise time something important had occurred in the case, as I did at 12:16 p.m., March 14, the moment Mom's vehicle crossed the border into Mexico, and it punched me in the stomach like a bully, reminding me of the work I had left to do. I could not rewrite history and I could not let go of it, as it was written, without an ending. I needed that ending desperately, so I dug in and worked harder.

Building relationships with experts in the media and law enforcement continued to be my focus. Pete's feature on Mom had sparked a lot of interest from other media outlets desiring anniversary update information on the case. Sherri and I teamed up as we had the previous year, speaking with reporters and giving on-camera interviews. Despite the negative statement by his boss at SDSO, Ray Henry stepped up for the family, speaking to media and releasing the video footage from the Wells Fargo ATM, where Mom was last seen in Vista, to the local television stations. Pete had become invested in helping our family in any way he could, going above and beyond his work on the news story.

As soon as I informed Pete that I had the border-crossing video, he took the tape to the Fox studio to see if his video guys could enhance it in some way and spent time analyzing it himself. He believed the video showed three people in Mom's van and offered to forward a copy to another of his close personal friends, LAPD Cold Case Detective, Cliff Shepard, and advised me to call

Shepard to discuss Mom's case, which I did. Cliff was a wealth of knowledge and suggestions, and he kindly offered to send the border-crossing video to the lab used by the Cold Case Unit. In early April, Pete emailed me to confirm that he had handed the tape over to Cliff. It would be a huge step forward in the case, because if we could see with whom Mom went to Mexico and discern whether or not she had been held against her will it would force SDSO and the FBI to focus their attention and resources on our investigation. It felt as though we were really close now to blowing the case wide open.

Our hard work and perseverance were beginning to pay off in other ways, too, with new developments occurring every week. Ray Henry called to inform me that SDSO would be handing Mom's landline records to Mexico within a few days, and almost simultaneously Miguel Ortiz called me, asking to set up a meeting with my sisters and me because Detectives Velez and Espinoza wanted us to look over the phone records with them to see if we could identify any familiar phone numbers.

I had written to my contact Adriana at Crime Stoppers San Diego, asking if they would consider featuring Mom's case on their website. To my complete surprise, Adriana emailed me back that our case was going to be one of two cases to be featured at the Crime Stoppers' Enough is Enough luncheon, an annual event honoring law enforcement officers from every agency in San Diego County, in late May and that there would be media invited to speak with us. Deb, Sher, Kim, and I spoke about what an incredible opportunity it was to bring more attention to Mom's murder, and we decided to substantially increase the reward we had been offering through Crime Stoppers since October from $1,000 to $10,000. We felt like it would be a good move to piggyback the media coverage we had gotten during the one-year anniversary with the announcement of the reward to give journalists new information to write and talk about. It never ceased to amaze me how vigilant my family had to be, and I had to be, to keep the focus on the investigation. I felt so fortunate to have the time and the resources to make that happen.

★   ★   ★

Near the end of April, I emailed Cliff and copied Pete, to ask for an update about the status of the video. Pete sent me a short response to let me know that Cliff was awaiting the verdict in the "Turner" trial, assuming I was aware of who he was referring to. On April 26 Cliff emailed to return the verdict on the border-crossing video, and it was not what I had hoped for:

> I apologize for taking so long to reply. I have been involved in a trial and haven't had much available time. I took the videotape to a law enforcement laboratory two days ago. The Tech looked at it and told me this: It is a copy. Which could be OK. But the problem with it is that there are 13 cameras. The tape records at approximately 30 frames per second. Each camera would record for 1 second, filling that frame of the videotape up with an image, with each camera doing so for the 13 seconds before repeating. When they copied the tape, they copied all 13 cameras views at one time, so that instead of having one image on a frame, there are. He said that enlarging it will not do very much. What he needs is an exact copy of the original tape. Then he could loop each camera station, and he could enlarge each frame so that detail will come out. Right now, the images on the copy are about 1/16th of the size of the originals. I know your family and the Mexican authorities have been working exceptionally hard, but do you think that you or another contact can emphasize how important an exact copy is, and convince them to provide one?

The news about the videotape really stung, it was not a dead end per se, but another mountain to climb, and I wasn't sure I had the strength to get up any more hills. I thanked Cliff for his help and assured him I would do everything possible to secure the original.

Four days later, I read the headlines on my newsfeed and was shocked to discover what the kind, mild-mannered and soft-spoken detective had been working on while helping out my family. Cliff made me feel as though he had all the time in the world to chat with me about Mom's case, and I had absolutely no clue he was in the middle of one of the biggest murder trials in the history of Los Angeles.

On April 30, 2007, Chester Dewayne Turner was convicted on eleven counts of murder, one of his victims an unborn child. Upon his conviction, Mr. Turner became known as the most prolific serial killer to date in Los Angeles County. Cliff, who was well known for his work using DNA evidence, had cleared a man, David Allen Jones, who had previously been charged with the murders and had served over ten years in prison for crimes he did not commit, and he built the case against Chester Turner. I sat slack-jawed at my laptop reading article after article about Cliff's work on the Turner case and had two thoughts—how lucky I was to have met him and how much I would like to have someone with Cliff's dedication and a detective of his caliber work on Mom's case.

In support of the great exposure *Crimestoppers* was giving Mom's case, my sisters and I bought a table at the Enough is Enough luncheon, hosted by the crime writer, Stephen J. Cannell, and invited Ray Henry and his superior, Dan Russell, to be our guests. As much as I had complained in the last year about what I saw as a lack of effort on our case, I had come to a place of understanding, and I was fully aware that there was only so much that

SDSO could do on our behalf because of the jurisdictional and logistical issues of a case that spanned two countries. Over lunch, I sat next to Ray and had the opportunity to show my appreciation for his interest in Mom's case.

"I really appreciate that you never make me feel bad about being the 'squeaky wheel' for my family," I said.

"You should never feel bad about calling, Lauri, you and your sisters are doing a wonderful thing. Let me tell you, I have been doing this job a long time, and I try to put myself in your shoes. It troubles me more when I don't hear from the family of a murder victim."

I nodded. "Thank you, Ray. I will keep calling because I am sure that I will not find the answers by myself."

I had no idea how prescient my words would be, because I would soon find a partner to help me dig for the truth.

FOURTEEN

Finding Candice

In June 2007 Mom's case was still parked in neutral, going nowhere in a hurry. Although there was a lot of activity surrounding the investigation in the first half of the year, and we had been hopeful about the border crossing video and Pete's show, no new leads had been generated from the Fox 11 news story in three months, and the border-crossing video appeared to be useless to investigators. On the positive side, relationships had been forged and were growing with detectives in Mexico and San Diego—something I hoped would pay off for us at some point.

The fear that there would be no closure for my family and me still loomed as a real possibility. Was I ready to give up? No, not even close. My sisters were counting on me to keep pushing for resolution, and I wanted to live up to their expectation. I also had some unfinished business with my own conscience and continued to struggle with questions about why and how Mom ended up in Mexico, murdered, and if I could have done anything to prevent it from happening by knowing her better, understanding her more, and being a real part of her life. There was a faceless murderer stalking my dreams, and I wanted desperately to find him or her so that I could properly grieve the loss of my mother's life and try to move on with my own. I just needed some serious help.

I had not watched much television in the last year because loud sounds still startled me, but a woman's voice pulled my attention from the pot I stirred in the kitchen, and when I looked across the island to the TV in the family room, her appearance drew me away to sit and listen. In some ways, she resembled my mother—a petite blonde with a short-cropped pixie haircut, dressed conservatively and professionally in a tailored women's suit. Her clear, dark blue eyes, which differed from my mom's brown, were as striking as her on-screen presence. Whoever she was, her posture told me she was confident in what she was saying. She was talking about a missing person's case, so I listened—hard.

Tanya Kach was a young woman who had been held against her will in a basement for ten years in McKeesport, Pennsylvania. Coincidentally, Miss Kach had been found the week of March 19, 2006, the same week Mom disappeared. "Candice DeLong, former FBI profiler" flashed across the screen as the woman commented on the sentencing of Chris J. Hose, the abductor and captor in the case. Ms. DeLong was outraged that he was sentenced to only five to fifteen years in prison for a crime he admitted to committing. She had been invited on air to offer her opinion about Miss Kach's mental state, given her years in captivity and the brevity of the sentence.

The interviewer added that prior to Ms. DeLong's service in the FBI, she had worked as a psychiatric nurse. Mom was fascinated by science, was well read on most of the subjects in current self-help literature, and had become an armchair psychologist of sorts, counseling anyone who would listen. *Mom would have loved to talk with this woman,* I thought. Hell, I wanted to talk to her. But how?

I spent the rest of the evening glued to my laptop Googling Candice DeLong. As soon as I woke, while my kids enjoyed one of their first sleep-ins of summer, I emailed Pete Noyes. I was excited to share the facts that I had learned about Candice and asked for his advice about the best way to contact her. Pete suggested, since she was the author of *Special Agent: My Life on the Front Lines as a Woman in the FBI,* I should try to reach her through her literary agent. After a quick round of breakfast slapped on the table for my kids, who were still so patient with their obsessed mother, I flew back to my laptop to find the name of Ms. DeLong's literary agent, hunt down an email address, and carefully compose a meaningful and convincing letter.

A quick search produced the name Elaine Koster, which when re-entered into the search engine returned pages of glowing endorsements from other notable authors she had worked with in her career, including Stephen King, Ken Follett, and Ms. Koster's most recent big-time discovery, Khaled Hosseini, who authored the blockbuster book "The Kite Runner." *Oh wow, with a client list like that, I will be lucky if this incredible woman has even a minute to look at my email,* I thought.

At 8:03 a.m. the following morning, I hit "send" on the letter I had labored and agonized over, and for the rest of the day could not bring myself to leave the house for fear of missing a response. Pete had shared so many great stories about cold cases solved years later through hard work and determination, and I was inspired and hopeful to be pursuing a new path in Mom's case. I must have checked my email fifty times, and then there it was at 2:37 p.m., an email from Elaine Koster. I had gotten lucky.

"Please contact Candice DeLong at . . ."

Oh my God, I did it!

I couldn't wait to contact Ms. DeLong, my fingers flew over the keys as I composed the following letter:

6/28/07

Dear Ms. DeLong,

I am writing to ask you for your assistance in my mother's murder investigation. I know that you are a published author and public speaker with a very full schedule, but wondered if, on occasion, you offered your expertise to families on a consulting basis.

My mother, Jane A. Kling was a business owner in Vista, California. On March 15, of last year, we reported her missing to the San Diego Sheriff's Office. Her body was found ten days later in a very remote part of Baja. She had been beaten and strangled, but was not sexually assaulted, although her clothing was partially removed. All of her personal possessions were found with her, including her purse and $300 cash was found in her socks next to her body. Her vehicle was also recovered from the scene. For your information, I have included a link below for a news piece/video produced by FOX LA.

We have 13 crime scene photos, actually taken by an American citizen, within hours of her death. My family and I would like to have them independently analyzed by a profiler because we believe they are very telling. It is our contention that she was not a victim of a random act of violence or a crime of opportunity as some in law enforcement would like for us to believe. The crime seems much more personal to all of us.

We are four daughters determined to find answers and would so appreciate your help in this matter. Please feel free to contact me with questions anytime.___-___-___ I thank you in advance for your assistance.

Kind regards,

Lauri Taylor

In my gut, I knew Candice would respond, but I didn't know why. To this point, my family and I had relied on traditional law enforcement, which was made up primarily of men. I couldn't help but think how much Mom would enjoy a little "Girl Power" in her corner. Thinking about it, I could hear Mom singing one of her favorite old Helen Reddy songs, "I Am Woman," which she regularly had blaring on the stereo throughout the house in 1972. Two days later, I received validation of my intuition and my first correspondence from Candice DeLong:

6/30/07

2:56 p.m.

I am so sorry about your mother. How shocking and sad. I don't know if I can help. I read the article. I have a few questions:

1: Have the authorities obtained her cell phone records? Gas receipts?

2. Was your mother seeing/dating anyone (man or woman)?

3. Could your mother have had a "secret" life that you didn't know about? Such as, a girlfriend?

4. Did she use drugs ever in the past 10 years?

5. What did the toxicology screen from the autopsy show?

6. Who stood to benefit from her death?

7. Do I understand the article correctly? Your mother was gone for 10 days then her freshly murdered body was found?

8. Who made the call (and to whom was the call made) that she had been murdered?

To answer these, just block highlight them, then click on "reply" then type in your answers next to each question.

Oh, one last question, how did you get my email address?

Sincerely,

Candice DeLong

Reading the last line of Candice's email made me smile. I had tracked down the personal email address of a former FBI agent, and even she wondered how I had been able to do it. Off and on throughout the day, I took my time to carefully respond to Candice's questions and tried to contain my excitement. Although grief still caused me to feel as though I was in the early stages of dementia—walking from room to room, forgetting what I had walked there for in the first place—my memory of the facts of Mom's case remained precise. When the house grew quiet later that night, I hammered out my response in short order:

6/30/07

10:14 p.m.

1: Have the authorities obtained her cell phone records? Gas receipts?

The San Diego Sheriff's Office and Mexican Authorities have my mother's cell records. There were no calls to or from Mexico. On the day before her disappearance there are seven calls to/from her cell phone, 4 are to voicemail with one of those calls lasting 13 minutes. She did not as a general rule check voicemail often and never for that length of time. The family obtained her financial records promptly and there was no bank card, credit card or gas card activity after March 13, the day before she disappeared.

2. Was your mother seeing/dating anyone (man or woman)?

Not that we are aware of. She was a widow for ten years and was reluctant (as far as we knew) to date because of her embarrassment about having a mastectomy and not having reconstructive surgery. She had a friendship of sorts with her landlord—his home was approximately 100 yards from hers. He came over to family events at her house such as Easter, occasionally. It did not appear to be a romantic relationship to the family. We know that they e-mailed some and there are a few calls to/from his number on her cell and business phones. Oddly though, when authorities asked about his relationship with my mother, he said it was "strictly landlord/tenant."

3. Could your mother have had a "secret" life that you didn't know about? Such as, a girlfriend?

Anything is certainly possible. My mother was married 4 times and seemed to love men, although, she always had girlfriends and enjoyed the company of women. In looking at her cell bill, it did not appear that there was someone that was calling her and she was calling back-not in the way you would call someone you are interested in. Also, she worked so many hours, all the people she worked with said she would never have had time to have a relationship.

4. Did she use drugs ever in the past 10 years?

This is an incredibly insightful question. . .My answer would have been no prior to my mother's death, but I have since learned that this was not the case. She was always one to grab an antibiotic or home remedy very quickly, but when her home was searched while she was missing, authorities found a large (300+pills) amount of Soma and a large amount of antacids in her bathroom. I now know that one of the side affects of overuse of Soma is digestive issues. She had to have her gall bladder removed a little over 6 months prior to her death. She ordered Soma through on line sources. The family was entirely unaware of her Soma use.

5. What did the toxicology screen from the autopsy show?

It showed that she had a prescriptive level of synthetic morphine in her system. Mexican authorities asked the family if we knew if she was suffering from a urinary tract infection because a mix of blood and urine were found in her van. No Soma was found in her purse or van.

6. Who stood to benefit from her death?

Absolutely no one. She owned/ran two consignment stores in Vista, California (a very odd place with a lot of drug users and a large homeless population) but she lived pay check to pay check and was helped out from time to time by her family. She rented the home she lived in, had no life insurance, pension or savings. The businesses were very tight financially—she had just opened a second store months earlier and had a big lease payment due. Many have opined that she was fleeing her business, but too many of her actions say she was not, including the fact that she made a business deposit the morning of March 14, hours before she disappeared. Why bother if you are leaving your business behind? All that being said, outsiders who did not know her financial state may have viewed her as someone who was well to do. She was good looking, dressed nicely and was well spoken.

7. Do I understand the article correctly? Your mother was gone for 10 days then her freshly murdered body was found?

Yes, she was missing for 10 days before her freshly murdered body was discovered in a very remote part of Mexico. SDSO informed the family on March 19 or 20, that my mother's van had crossed the border at Calexico/Mexicali at a little after noon on March 14. Exact time of death is an issue, but based on what we were told by locals about the area, we believe she died late March 23 or early 24. There is a big coyote/wild dog population in the area and we were told that if her body had been there very long, it would have been consumed. Also, the photos that we have, that were taken by an American, seem to confirm that she had not been deceased a long time. In comparison, Polaroids taken approximately 10-12 hours later by Mexican authorities at the scene show changes in her facial features looking as though rigor mortis had begun to set in.

8. Who made the call (and to whom was the call made) that she had been murdered?

My eldest sister Debbie received a call from the Ministerio Público in San Felipe on March 25 at 1:30 in the afternoon.

The District Attorney there, Jorge Silva, called her personally. Debbie's phone number was found in Mom's purse on her business card. He told her that our mother had died under unusual circumstances and that we needed to come the following day to identify and claim her body.

Candice, thank you so very much for taking the time to answer my e-mail and for your kind words. I got your e-mail address from Elaine Koster. I knew that you were published, so I sent her an e-mail telling her that I would like to contact you to inquire about reviewing the crime scene photos of my mother's case. I hope that I have not intruded on your privacy by e-mailing you at this address.

We may have jurisdictional issues, language barriers and a case that is growing colder by the minute, but my sisters and I are still hopeful. I thank you for taking the time to look at my responses and would be happy to provide additional information, if appropriate. Take care.

All my best,

Lauri Taylor

Candice began an endless stream of inquiry and I was thrilled she was asking me. The more she asked, the more detail I provided. I could feel her becoming invested in Mom's story with each thoughtful comment and carefully asked question. She asked me about elements of the case that no other member of law enforcement had asked before, which solidified her expert status in my mind and made me feel like an authority on Mom's case. We exchanged several more emails over the course of two days; then our correspondence stopped for the Fourth of July holiday. I began to grow nervous that Candice had lost interest. On the tenth, I couldn't wait another minute or day longer and decided to write to tell Candice exactly why I needed her help:

7/10/07

7:05pm

Dear Candice,

I hope you enjoyed a great 4th of July holiday! I wanted to reconnect with you about my mother's case and tell you how much I appreciated your time last week. I also wanted to let you know why we need your help.

Over the course of the last year, we have struggled to keep the San Diego Sheriff's Office involved in our case. Quite simply, the lead detective developed a theory about my mother's death, and did not pursue any investigation beyond that. They told us the murder occurred in Mexico, therefore it is Mexico's case, despite the fact that the last known person my mother was seen with in Mexico was said to be American. They believed that my mother was in a compromised mental state because of the Soma, went to Mexico on her own (we have an official request in to Mexico City for video tape from Mexicali that may show Mom's van crossing the border with two other individuals), got stuck in a remote area and was beaten and strangled by a stranger. They have implied Mexican police conspiracy (one would think if they were conspiring to cover up a homicide that my mother's death would have been ruled something different). Their cooperation with Mexico has been limited and strained, while the family's relationship with Mexico is very good.

In October, without a single individual in the US having been questioned by SDSO since she was missing, they closed her case. My sisters and I pursued a political course of action, were granted a meeting with the Undersheriff of San Diego, Bill Gore (former FBI), and following our appeal and presentation of facts, our case was re-opened. The two lead detectives in our case were re-assigned. The new Sgt. in charge has been much more responsive and communicative with our family. Although they have yet to question anyone in Mom's case, we are very slowly moving toward that (we finally got Mom's detailed landline records after a year of requests).

As determined and resourceful as my sisters and I may be, we do not have the expertise or training necessary to drive this investigation. We just don't know what questions need to be asked next. Our mother raised us to have great trust and respect for law enforcement; unfortunately, we have learned, that we must be the "squeaky wheel" for our case to get the attention it deserves. To that end, we need help in coordinating the investigation between Mexico and the US, in developing and exploring all possible theories and suspects and for someone to look at the totality of our evidence and help to develop a plan to move forward and fully investigate this case.

The reason I wanted you to look at our crime scene photos (and any other evidence) was to see if you could determine anything about our suspect. Obviously, a determination of stranger vs. acquaintance suspect pool could put pressure on SDSO to investigate on this side of the border. Because our Undersheriff is former FBI, I believe a detailed assessment by a fellow agent would carry great weight with him.

Please let me know your thoughts when you have a moment and, as always, I thank you for your time.

Sincerely yours,

Lauri Taylor

Candice's response three hours later left me giddy and unable to sleep. *Maybe this is finally it—the breakthrough we need,* I thought:

7/10/08

10:01pm

Okay, let's talk Thursday. I have thought a/b your mother's murder a lot. It does not surprise me that SDSO is not pursuing this, and I have no reason to believe that Mexico will do anything out of their way to solve it either. But I must tell you that I do not do private investigating (or what I call "footwork" on cases) I only consult. also, you need to understand that although my expertise is in crimes of interpersonal violence, I am not always correct. There are a lot of unknowns in some murders and in those cases I can only offer my best opinion. My opinion, however, is based on 35 years of experience, both clinical and as an FBI profiler. I take on very few private cases because, quite frankly, I don't need the aggravation or stress. Families/clients sometimes don't like my opinion if it's not the same one they had in mind. But you seem very intelligent and reasonable, so let's talk about how I *might* be of assistance.

When is a good time for you? Anytime after 10:00 am is good for me.

Candice DeLong

By the next morning, Candice and I had made plans to talk on Thursday, July 12 at 11:00 am, and suddenly the sense of overwhelming pride I had worn for the past couple of weeks was traded in for a fresh set of anxiety handcuffs. *Oh my God, how will I convince her to take our case? What was I thinking? What does it even cost to hire a former FBI profiler?* The naysayer chorus played in my head and my stomach turned.

I walked straight to my closet, dug out my exercise clothes, and yelled down the hall to the kids. "I'm going to do the hills, be back in about an hour!"

Laced up and ready to sweat, I hit the pavement of the cul-de-sac hard with my first step off the driveway. The hills had been a great escape for me over the last several months, as I battled the effects of lingering depression with exercise and tried not to completely obsess about Mom's case—but in point of fact, I was only trading one obsessive compulsive behavior for another. When I needed it, however, exercise did help me to stop patterns of negative thinking. On my walks, I tried to spend as much time as possible charging uphill, causing my heart rate to soar, and instead of thinking about my fears, I focused on counting each step in eight counts as I had when I choreographed routines as a pompom girl at SMU. *One, two, three, four, five, six, seven, eight, one, two, three, four, five, six, seven, eight.* Sometimes I would go out at night alone even though the thought of what lurked in the shadows scared the hell out of me. I had to face my fears now, stare them down, or they would get the better of me.

On Thursday, July 12, I phoned Candice. We spoke for over an hour and had very quick rapport. My fears were laid to rest by her funny, dry humor, as we shared personal background information and she told me a little about her life as a psychiatric nurse prior to her quest to become an FBI agent. She was fascinating and personable at the same time, and she was complimentary about what my family had accomplished in Mom's case so far. But she told me that a recent experience had negatively affected how she felt about consulting work, and she shared her concerns with me.

A family, much like my own, had asked her for help. Candice worked many hours on their behalf and delivered a concise opinion about their case. The family did not like the conclusions that she had drawn and refused to pay the rather large sum of money they owed her. I could hear the slight hesitation in her voice when we talked about the possibility of her working with me. Despite the fact that it was not at all in my nature to press people for anything, I had developed some skills in the last year, and I knew this was a do or die moment in our conversation, so I drew in a deep breath and dove in.

"As you know, I have no training in law enforcement and believe I have taken my mom's case as far as I can. I want desperately to give my family closure, some sort of answer about what happened to our mother, even if it is your best guess, based on your years of experience and training. You are the expert here and I promise you, I will not question your conclusion."

"Ok, I'll do it," she said.

What does it cost to hire a former FBI agent? A lot. But I didn't care. I would have paid anything. I didn't want anyone to tell me no, so I didn't ask anyone's permission. I hired Candice on the spot.

FIFTEEN

What to Feed an FBI Profiler

My sisters had trusted me to this point in the case and I felt like I could fly on my own, as long as I kept them in the loop. I had not asked for anyone's permission or approval, neither my husband's nor my sisters', to find or hire Candice, which was not my normal modus operandi. The more I ventured out on my own, the more confident I became in my ability to lead Mom's investigation, finding a voice I did not know I had in the process. I had earned a new level of respect from my family, the male detectives, and for myself, and I knew my mother would be wholly proud of this incarnation of me, which was heartening.

When she was younger, Mom worked in a male-dominated culture, the banking industry, and reveled in the fact that she had not only broken into it, but had risen to its highest ranks. Now I was experiencing something similar. Ray Henry was becoming more communicative and validating, and as a result, SDSO began to interact with the California Department of Justice investigators and the PGJE in Ensenada, often with me as a conduit to actively investigate Mom's case. Miguel Ortiz continued to be a loyal supporter, sharing calls and emails with me, showing his trust at every turn. The addition of Candice to the team made me feel as though the outcome of the case truly rested in my hands, which was exhilarating and frightening at the same time, but a responsibility that I suddenly felt entirely capable of managing.

The synchronicity of seeing Candice on television, contacting her agent, and having her agree to work with me in the short span of three weeks, left me with the sense that we were intended to meet and work together. I had a gut feeling about contacting her, and I went for it. Candice's funny, dry, and sarcastic personality was a breath of fresh air to me, but she also brought a hefty dose of empathy and expertise. We emailed, texted, and chatted often, sharing details of the case and tidbits about ourselves, and we quickly built a great working relationship. In response to my question of whether I should keep anyone on stand-by for the day of our meeting, Candice wrote:

> That's an excellent question, and very foresighted of you, but I'm not surprised. I mean after all, this is Lauri we're talking about! I think I would have enjoyed working with you. Many of my colleagues were pretty lazy and unimaginative. That said, let's just keep it you and me for now.
>
> I think that after several hours with you I will have a very long list of things that need to be done or redone, and I can always call people later.
>
> As for keeping someone on stand-by, tell me, do you have faith in your PI? Is this the same one that you've always had? Is he a retired FBI agent? The reason I ask is, I find that a lot of PIs (as well as sworn officers), are threatened by my presence in a case. They tend to get very defensive if they haven't "solved" the case. As for me being an FBI profiler, well, many "badges of a lesser God" (as I call them) simply write off what I do as hocus-pocus nonsense. But actually, it isn't the only tool I use to investigate a crime; it's just one tool. I've been involved or profiled hundreds of murders while most FBI agents never even investigate one murder in their entire career. Something to bear in mind: Cops/agents are very competitive and

highly territorial, much like river hippos. They charge and attack if they even perceive a threat, and look pretty funny while doing so. But if you *REALLY* want to see a good "my badge is bigger than your badge" battle, get 2 FBI profilers or profiler wanna-be(s) in a room and, oh, wait! I forgot, there *is* no room big enough for 2 FBI profilers to occupy! ☺.

In our early conversations, Candice had told me, "Talking with you is like talking with another profiler." I was floored and proud, and continued to hold my self-doubt at bay, at least for the moment. If Candice believed this about me, then I could believe it about myself, a feeling that grew within me as we arranged our first face-to-face meeting. As luck would have it, Candice already had plans to fly to Los Angeles to do an interview for MSNBC in a few weeks. We confirmed by email that Candice would arrive at John Wayne Airport on Thursday, August 2, 2007, and stay locally to prep for her segment, "The Mind of Manson" with Keith Morrison, which was scheduled to film on Friday in Los Angeles. Candice explained that she had been hired to analyze a *Today Show* prison interview of Charles Manson that had aired twenty years earlier, and to give her professional observations of the cult murderer.

I jumped on amazon.com and had a copy of Candice's book, *Special Agent: My Life on the Front Lines as a Woman in the FBI*, sent overnight so I could learn everything possible about her career before her arrival, and I devoured it in a day. Fascinated by the incredible cases she had worked, from the Unabomber to the Tylenol murders, her law enforcement pedigree was stellar. Candice's fit image, complete with shoulder holster and gun, commanded my attention from the cover of the book. Close-cropped dark hair, crystal blue eyes, and high cheek bones gave Candice the appearance of one of my cop show idols, but she was real, and she was coming to *my house* on Saturday! *Omg, what do I feed an FBI profiler?* I thought.

When I pulled in under the covered entrance to the Marriott hotel, a tiny blonde woman, dressed professionally in a taupe suit jacket with slacks and heels, waved me down as I nearly drove past. Slamming on the brake, I screeched to a stop. She smiled broadly through the window at me, and I knew it was her. All that reading had left me with a larger than life image of Candice as a towering, Wonder Woman-like figure, despite the fact that the book had described her as petite and had shown her as a brunette.

"Hi, Lauri?" Candice asked, through the open window, jumping into the front seat of my SUV, when I simply nodded, yes, because I was suddenly speechless.

★ ★ ★

Mercifully, Candice recognized my complete state of awe and began to chat the second she buckled herself into the seat, breaking the ice, and she kindly asked me questions throughout the fifteen minute drive to my house. We spent the next seven hours parked at my kitchen table in deep discussion, taking only a short break for lunch without even a minute of silence passing between us.

We were both beat up and starving by the end of the day. During breaks in conversation about the case, we had discovered that we were both foodies and loved wine. I asked Candice if I could treat her to a nice dinner before she returned to her hotel, which she gladly accepted. We headed back to the Ruth Chris steakhouse and squeezed into two seats at the corner of the long wooden bar as the restaurant bustled with Saturday night clientele, and we waited for our table. Above the hum of the crowd, Candice ordered a martini and I ordered a glass of wine, and we began to chat about our favorite foods and favorite restaurants.

"Have you ever been to Boulevard Restaurant? It's near the ferry building." I asked, sipping on my glass of Cabernet.

"I have; it's a beautiful spot and the food is spectacular," she said.

"I have some great memories of Boulevard. I surprised Rick for his fortieth birthday. A group of his college friends flew in from Kansas to celebrate for the weekend. We also ate there with friends during the OJ Bronco chase."

"Oh, don't get me started on OJ," Candice laughed.

"Really? I was fascinated by that case and watched every minute of the television coverage." I didn't bother telling her that I had read every book written about the case. "Do you have an opinion or theory?"

Candice let out a low chuckle and grinned, and I laughed, too. *I suppose that was a silly question to ask an FBI profiler who is featured regularly on television to offer her expert opinion.* Candice was just beginning to share her insight about the forensic aspects of the OJ case when a large gentleman slouching on the stool to my right, whose Tommy Bahama shirt hung awkwardly, barely covering the waistband of his slacks, scooted his chair towards me.

"OJ didn't do it," he bellowed at Candice and me. The wafting smell of whiskey trailing his words, the inebriated stranger seemed unconcerned about his intrusion of our private conversation. Apparently he missed the totally aghast expressions on our faces, as well, and proceeded to churn out his opinion of the facts of the case. Candice very coolly picked up her martini and sipped, sneaking a wink at me over the brim of the crystal glass, while graciously feigning interest in his diatribe. She nodded and smiled at our uninvited guest as I sat sandwiched between them. Every so often she would nod or simply say "aha," *This guy has absolutely no clue who he is talking to,* I thought, smiling. Thankfully the bartender interrupted and told Candice and me that our table was ready. We quickly settled up our tab, and followed the hostess who directed us to our booth and handed us each a menu. As soon she was out of earshot, Candice looked at me and we broke out in laughter.

"You were so kind not to humiliate him back there," I said.

"Remember, we do not engage amateurs, especially not drunk ones, in those types of discussions. We leave that to the professionals," she said, lifting her glass to toast me.

"Cheers," I said, lifting my glass to meet hers, and swallowed the lump that had sprung up in my throat.

I'm not sure Candice knew how much her comment meant to me (although she *was* a psych nurse for twenty years, so she probably did), but it was the ultimate validation of the work I had done on Mom's case so far and made me feel incredibly proud. She truly made me feel like we were going to be partners in the investigation.

In the weeks after our first meeting, I was so inspired by Candice's kind words and confidence in me, I could hardly wait to jump back into the case. My life and my kids' lives had been completely upended over the last year and a half, and I hoped that hiring Candice would be the answer to our prayers. Candice encouraged me to reevaluate the evidence that I had access to, including Karla Nelson's photos, files, and phone records, and to continue to hammer law enforcement for the information we still did not have—a copy of Mom's autopsy, the toxicology reports, and Mexico's crime scene photos.

If I was going to be a real investigator, examining evidence was part of my job description, and I wanted to show Candice that her confidence in me was not misplaced. If she believed I was up to the task of working this investigation *with* her, then I would work it. My goal was to find some piece of evidence that would compel San Diego Sheriff's Office and/or the FBI to pursue leads and more interviews in the United States. The fact that Mom had been seen with an English-speaking woman in San Felipe had us convinced that the crime could have started on the US side of the border.

It took me a week to get up the nerve to *really* look at Karla Nelson's photos. Rick, Clark, and Katy were with friends at a Friday night Angel's baseball playoff game, normally one of my very favorite activities, but I chose to stay behind to do some investigative work while the house was empty. I would be able to blow up and print out the photos without worrying that the kid's would accidentally see the frightening pictures of their grandmother. Our printer was in the office/playroom upstairs where they watched television, studied, and played video games and I didn't want to take that risk.

To say that I am technologically challenged is only a slight exaggeration of the truth. In my defense, I had gotten a new laptop and was not completely familiar with how to use Photoshop, but eventually zeroed in on the one program feature I needed for my work: the zoom. I clicked on picture number 1, and steeled myself for the shock that I was sure would come as the image of Mom's body lying in the dirt filled my screen. My heart ached, and I wanted to cry, but this wasn't the time; I had investigating to do before my kids got home. Picture number 1 was taken from a distance, facing east, and even when blown up to the fullest setting, it was difficult to see anything significant. Pictures 5 through 9, were thankfully, not pictures of Mom's body. They were shots of items from around the scene including Mom's shoes, a black jacket, envelopes that appeared to be bank statements strewn about under a shrub, and Mom's purse were photographed in the area near where her body was found.

By the time I had gotten to Picture 13, the last of the Karla Nelson photos, I felt pretty numb to the effects of seeing Mom's corpse up close, and 13 was the only photo taken from a relatively close distance, from below Mom's body near her feet. I began to zoom in, searching the sand, her feet, the debris on her sweats, and every inch of Mom's body. I had zoomed in as far as Photoshop would allow me to, which made the images a bit fuzzy. When I reached Mom's arms I paused, struck by the odd scabbing in a zigzag pattern on her lower forearm. It didn't appear to be scratch marks, but could be some other kind of defense wound. I had recently learned about ligature marks—the kind of wound that results from being bound with a rope or cord. *What if this is a ligature mark? What if I have found the key to Mom's case?* I thought.

I texted Candice immediately and she answered me back right away, even though she was just finishing dinner and a glass of wine. She jumped on her computer so we could look at the photos at the same time.

"A ligature means she was being held against her will," Candice reminded me. "Since there were no other torture marks on her body, whoever was holding her was not doing it for sadistic pleasure, but rather for strictly practical reasons, i.e., to keep her with him until he was ready to kill her."

Candice's words sent a chill up my spine, and the thought sickened me.

"Are you okay, Lauri?" she asked, never losing sight that we were talking about my mother.

"I'm good, thanks. Let's keep going," I said.

Candice and I continued to look through all the photos, speculating about lividity, which is the natural settling of blood in a corpse post mortem, the bruising around Mom's neck, the place in the sand where her feet appeared to have dug in. It was nearly 11:00 and Rick and the kids would be coming home soon.

Candice and I ended our call and agreed to talk again soon. But as soon as the line went dead, it was as if the curtain had been pulled back, exposing the imposter daughter, who had been posing as an investigator, just like when Dorothy exposed the Wizard, and I felt raw and battered.

★ ★ ★

My family needed closure so that we could begin to rebuild our lives and we needed a break from the stress of the investigation. Closure wasn't happening anytime soon, so we focused on taking a break. Rick and I took the kids on a trip to Europe for Clark's 16th birthday and started plans to put a pool in our backyard so that Clark and Katy would have a place to socialize with friends at home. I wanted them close to me, close to home, because I so feared the unpredictability of the world. Undertaking a major construction project in order to accomplish this goal seemed totally reasonable to me at the time.

Despite the fact that I was traveling with my kids while we vacationed in Ireland, I became very anxious and thought that it might be because I felt out of touch with the ongoing case. When my jet lag compounded my anxiety and I could not sleep, I emailed Ray Henry from the hotel bathroom while my family slept in the other room. Ray was true to his word and emailed back that he had assigned a cold case investigator, Tommy Nash, to the investigation, whom he was preparing to brief about the details of the case to date. Sgt. Henry was also making arrangements for one of the top polygraph technicians in San Diego to question Sylvia Murphy in early September and would invite Mexican detectives to be present during the questioning. This was a huge step forward in the case because it indicated there would be real cooperation between Mexico and the United States. Ray Henry had heard me when I asked him to investigate Sylvia Murphy, if for no other reason than to eliminate her as a person of interest.

The Sergeant in Charge of Homicide surprised me further when he called me personally following Sylvia's interview to share the results of the polygraph with me.

Ray shared with me that the officer administering the polygraph believed Sylvia had been truthful in answering all of the questions. Although he was comfortable with me sharing the information with Candice, he would prefer for me not to share the results with my sisters. I didn't ask Ray why he made this request, because I felt privileged that he was sharing it at all, but my guess was that Ray was concerned the information could somehow get back to Sylvia.

My heart sank because it had taken a year and a half of nearly constant requests to persuade SDSO to conduct that interview with Sylvia and it was a total dead end. I agreed to Sgt. Henry's request to keep the news to myself, feeling like I had been granted access to the private club. But at the same time, I felt as though I was breaking the pact I had made with my sisters. We had promised one another that we would stick together throughout this tragedy, and now I was keeping information from them and stepping out on my own.

I emailed Candice to tell her about my phone call from Ray Henry regarding Sylvia's polygraph, and about my disappointment in the results. We were at a standstill, and Sylvia's interview seemed to take the wind out of the sails for SDSO to investigate people of interest in the United States. Candice agreed that without any evidence pointing to the crime having begun in the US or Mom being held against her will, SDSO would not feel obligated to investigate.

"We need autopsy photos, Lauri." Candice said. "I hope they exist."

Me too, I thought.

As had begun to be our pattern, a conversation with Candice always inspired me to go back to the case, back to digging. So that's what I did.

One of the odd markings on Mom's body that was still yet to be explained had been pointed out by one of Sherri's close friends, Megan, who had been very helpful to our family when Mom disappeared. The two red, slightly smaller than dime-size marks on Mom's lower abdomen were spaced about an inch or so apart. Megan, who had no special training, had suggested they looked like taser marks. If I could prove that the spots on Mom's stomach were taser marks, then I hoped *someone* in law enforcement would really jump on Mom's case.

One afternoon while Clark was at golf and Katy was upstairs playing a video game with a friend, I sat at my defacto desk at the kitchen table, Googled, "Taser Marks" and clicked "images" so that I had something to compare to the marks on Mom's stomach. The montage of body parts, bruised flesh and corpses sickened me, but what upset and confused me the most was that the sweet face of JonBenet Ramsey was interspersed amongst these horrible images. I clicked on several pictures that had markings that looked similar to Mom's and it seemed to me the taser theory might be plausible. I chose another taser image and clicked, gasping when JonBenet's dead body filled my screen, nearly throwing up. I quickly closed the window and, devastated, began to cry.

Very soon after our family was notified that Mom had been murdered, I began to feel part of a strange club—the violent crime victims' club. I had always felt heartbroken and empathetic for families whose loved ones were victims of murder, such as Nicole Brown's family, Natalee Holloway's family, Samantha Runion's family, and JonBenet Ramsey's family, and now I felt like I could relate to them on a much deeper level and understand their pain better.

Not only was I soaking in terrible guilt because it felt as though I had violated the Ramsey family's right to privacy by viewing such a personal photograph, I agonized for her poor mother over the guilt she must have felt about not being able to protect her little girl. It was also an awful reminder that some cases are just never solved, which hit too close to home and sent me back on the search for clues from the evidence I had in my possession.

Sherri had recently entrusted me with a tub of paperwork and other items from Mom's home and desk at work. Digging through it one afternoon in October, I came across Mom's large white desk calendar, unfolded it and laid it on my kitchen table. I started at the top and worked my way down the document, trying to put a fresh set of eyes on every item written on each square. There was very little written on the calendar, but seeing Mom's signature loopy, feminine, handwriting made me wistful. Down towards the bottom right-hand side of the page though, something was scribbled sideways and upside down. I turned the large sheet of paper around to get a better look. *Oh my God*, I thought, *this could finally be it!*

It was someone's email address but the username is what got me: Mulege22. Mulege was a city in Baja, much farther south than Puertecitos, but on the same side of the peninsula on the Sea of Cortez. I had spent much of the summer on Baja travel blogs and had researched news stories in Mexico to determine if there were cases similar to Mom's in other areas of Baja. Otherwise, I would not have been familiar with the city of Mulege. I had just stumbled upon the only piece of evidence that linked Mom to Mexico; previously, law enforcement had not found any recent connection. I called Ray Henry immediately to inform him of my discovery and he asked me to make a copy and overnight it to him.

"We'll look into it for you, Lauri," he promised.

Then I called Candice, and she applauded me for my sleuthing. We began to talk seriously about what our next move would be with SDSO's sudden cooling off on the case. Candice felt as though we should have another expert look at the crime scene photos and suggested a close personal friend and colleague of hers who, she said, "has been in the business a long time."

"That would be incredible." I said.

"My colleague is Dr. Michael Baden . . . you may have heard of him," she said.

I almost fell out of my chair, but remained calm. "Yes, I have heard of him," I said, trying to sound casual.

Dr. Michael Baden was not just any doctor; he happened to be the leading forensic pathologist in the country. He was regularly consulted as an expert witness on high-profile deaths, such as Nicole Brown Simpson and John Belushi, and appeared as a regular guest expert on all the news shows. Dr. Baden lived in New York, where Candice loved to travel around the holidays. She scheduled an appointment to meet with him in early December. I put a notebook together filled with all the information and evidence I had compiled on Mom's case. Candice joked that the notebook was "bureau-worthy," which of course made me proud and hopeful that a break in the case would come as a result of it.

On December 12, 2007, I pulled into a parking space at the outlet mall, just outside of Palm Springs, California. I was with my girlfriends, who had joined me there to see Kimi's client, Tony Orlando, perform at the Morongo Casino later that night. My phone rang just as I turned off the car. It was Candice, and so naturally I answered.

"Can you hold on a moment?" I asked, motioning for the girls to get started shopping without me.

"Hey, Lauri," she asked, "Can you talk?"

"Yes, I can. I'm by myself now. Go ahead." I said, reaching into the glove box for something to write on, and grabbed a stack of 3 × 5 cards and a pen so I could take notes.

Candice dove right in to Dr. Baden's remarks about the evidence we had sent. There wasn't much for me to take notes on. Dr. Baden hadn't found anything conclusive – he was not convinced that what I had seen in photo #13 was a ligature mark. Candice reminded me that we should focus on acquiring the autopsy photos and Mom's van, and be open to all possibilities. My heart sank, the tears of disappointment welling up, and I think I forgot to breathe; my head swirled, and I felt light-headed. I had so hoped for something more, for an ending, but Candice was telling me I needed to get back to work on the case. *I'll do that*, I thought, *just as soon as I scrape what's left of me up off of the floor.*

Staring down at the few words I had written during our conversation, I breathed deeply, filling my chest and shuffled the small stack of cards I held in my hands. I turned them over one by one, and caught my breath, reading words that I had not written myself. In my haste, I had grabbed my son's Spanish vocabulary flash cards. Written in pencil across each card, in Clark's blocky printing were, the words "brazo, cabeza, dientes—arm, head and teeth." No matter how hard I had tried to keep Mom's case separate from our life or to personally be done with looking at body parts, the universe continued to remind me that the investigation had woven itself into the fabric of our life, and that I was far from being done investigating body parts in Mexico.

SIXTEEN

El Muerto

There was a lot more to pray about than there was to toast to on New Year's Eve of 2007. We spent time over the Christmas break visiting Grandma Mary at the hospital and I was fairly certain that it would be the last time Clark, Katy, and I would see my sweet mother-in-law, as her health was declining quickly. Rick was juggling negotiations with his new employer and remained in constant contact with his brother, Rocky, about Mary's illness. My kid's were struggling with losing their beloved grandma and with Rick's recent decision to leave his job in January and commute full time to the East Coast, a decision which would mean he would not be at home as much, and which would mean they would no longer be "Toshiba kids." They had come to adore the tightly knit community of families whose parents worked at the company and with whom we spent a great deal of our social time.

As for me, I was thoroughly tapped out. Dr. Baden's opinion about Mom's case had left me completely at a loss, but figuring out how to move the case forward when there seemed nowhere else to go, was definitely not a priority. With so much in our life proving to be unpredictable and unsettling, I had no energy for it.

Bright spots and happy moments were few and far between during those months.

A tiny bright spot did occur though when I received a kind and heartfelt New Year's Day email from Miguel Ortiz.

First of all, i hope you had a very great CHRISMAS, with your love ones, and of course BEST WISHES FOR 2008, i want to apollogise (hope thats spelld correctly), for all the inconviniens that dealling with the case, because, some infromation, and articles, were not send to the agents in the US, i dont have an idea of the reasons that the coaporation has stopt all of a sudent, this is not a justification, but, there were a lot of CHANGES, in the structure of the DISTRICT ATTORNES offices, and state POLICE, in the past months, i my self, a couple of days a go, i was sent to ROSARITO B.C., for un noun reasons, and i dont now if ill be back in Ensenada any time soon, all i can tell you is that therese now BOSSES in the state captital and there taking drastic discsions, i hope this will be for the best interes of our society and of course in resolving your case, i felt we got on the right track, with the new agents from the US, and the only thing i can tell you is keep insisting with the new people, so the case keeps going the right way, once again i apolligise, for not beeing hable to move the case any futher, in that i nou i failed you, and i am very sorry, still i want you to now that if theres any thing i can help you with, ill do wathevers in my hands to HELP You, Consider me a mexican friend you can count on.

MIGUEL ORTIZ

I was thankful I could count on Miguel to help where he could, but was also keenly aware that there was only so much he could do in his position in Mexico, and one misstep could not only cost him his livelihood but possibly his life. It would be a huge violation of his job to be sharing information with the family of the victim in a criminal case, particular a family that wasn't Mexican. Because of the drug cartels and corruption at all levels, working in law enforcement in Mexico was a very dangerous job. Being one of the good guys, a person who operated with the utmost integrity, was even harder, but Miguel Ortiz was most definitely a good guy. I emailed him back and thanked him for his dedication to my mother's case and for his friendship, and let him know I would be calling on him in the New Year. My own life was treacherous to negotiate right now but his was treacherous on a completely different level.

We came home from our sad visit to Kansas and the kids started back at school. Two weeks later, Rick got the call that Mary was failing. I stayed home to shepherd the kids through the start of the new semester and Rick flew back to be at his mother's side. On January 16, 2008, Rick's birthday, Rick called to tell me that Grandma Mary had passed away.

"Mom just died," Rick choked out through his tears.

"Oh my God," I choked out through my own, "I am so sorry. Where are you, are you okay?"

"I walked outside to call you. Rocky, Debbie, and I were there with her. Mom's breathing changed and then she just stopped."

I truly loved Mary and I was confident she loved me, and was incredibly sad that I could not be there with Rick, his brother Rocky, and my sister-in-law Debbie at Mary's bedside, but I was so thankful for them to be there with their mother. Mary deserved that blessing, and they deserved it, too. I would have given anything to have had a moment like that with my own mother—to have been able to tell her, "Thank you for all that you taught me, you are an amazing woman whom I have admired for your courage and determination, and I love you so very much."

Clark and Katy took the passing of their second grandmother really hard. She had been nothing but pure unconditional love and joy to them, to all of us. Two days later, we flew to Kansas to meet Rick to attend Mary's funeral and on a frigid and icy winter day, we laid Mary to rest.

Our lives, however, were still anything but restful. We came home and Rick began his new job. It was a good career move for him, and he always worked hard to support our family, but having him gone four to five days a week was a blow. The investigation had taken a toll on us, too and I began to feel disconnected from him. Then on top of all that, Clark, who was a sophomore in high school and had never been in a minute of trouble before, got into his first fight ever. My life that had once been so tame and predictable felt like it was spinning out of control.

It was a difficult time. One night, gasping for air, my heart pounding in my chest, uncontrollably, I sat straight up in bed to try to catch my breath. Everything was pitch black, save for the illuminated numbers on the cable box that read, 2:30 am. Damp and cold, drenched in sweat and tears, I shivered, and pulled my comforter up under my chin. Clutching the covers, I laid my head back on the pillow and opened my mouth, heaving in a deep breath, and felt my heart rate begin to slow. *I am in my room, I'm fine, I'm fine, I'm fine.* I thought, trying to convince myself. I had grown accustomed to nightmares. One in particular I had quite frequently over the years since Mom's death. The picture of Mom's last stand on that stretch of desert wash was seared into my brain. She fought for her life, clawing, wrestling, and struggling in the darkness, the sound of angry waves crashing on the shore of the Sea of Cortez a few hundred yards away muffled the sound of the blows to her body and her screams in the night. Thankfully, that dream had tapered off in regularity and only seemed to stalk me when I was closely involved in examining or discussing evidence in the case.

The dream I had just awakened to, though, was a different one. It was one that I had dreamed quite often, back when I was a child in elementary school. An enormous tidal wave was coming.

As the towering wall of water loomed ominously in the distance, I stood alone on the shore, paralyzed by my fear, powerless to escape it. My little feet, were sunk deeply into the wet, cold sand that engulfed them tightly around my ankles, and it felt as though I were wearing cement boots. While I waited helplessly for my fate on the shoreline, I imagined myself being held under water by the force of the crushing wave and wondered how long I would remain conscious, fully aware that I would suffocate before I actually died. That is the part that haunted me most—the knowing I was going to die.

It did not take a great stretch of my imagination to draw the similarities between what I was experiencing in my nightmare as a reflection of what I envisioned had happened to my mom, but there was more to it. This dream was about me—my fear, and my feelings of utter powerlessness about the course of my life and facing it all alone.

By the end of February, there had been very little movement on the investigation. Eduardo Reyes, who had been such a support at Cal DOJ, had been transferred to another department and was no longer a resource for me there. Candice was busy traveling for a new television show and shared with me that she would be tied up with filming until May. I tried not to panic, but obsessed that interest in the case was dwindling, and I decided it was time for me to stir the pot, again.

I phoned the US Consulate in Mexico to request an original copy of the official video of Mom's border crossing and asked for their help in trying to track down the van. I created a new email account, and without asking permission of Ray or anyone else in charge of the investigation, sent an email to "Mulege22," telling them about my mom and asking for a response. This was a reckless act, because the owner of the screen name "Mulege22" was still a suspect in the case. Nothing happened on either front. I received no help from the consulate and no reply to my email.

I dreaded March, and all the memories associated with it, but I was desperate for joy and decided the only way to guarantee it was to manufacture it myself. I began to hunt for a dog. My friends and family thought I was out of my mind, and I was—with grief, and sorrow and sadness, and anxiety—but I was completely cognizant of what I was doing when I found Katy's 14th birthday present online: a precious, fluffy, cream- colored Labrador puppy, who had been born on January 16th, the day Grandma Mary passed away. Rick, Katy, her friend Ashley, and I drove two hours to the breeder to pick up the plump, female fur ball, which Katy named Bella. She was pure love, like all babies are, and just what the doctor had ordered.

The second anniversary of Mom's death came with my usual correspondence to law enforcement to remind them that our case was still unsolved, as if they could have forgotten since I emailed them last month. The flurry of media that had surrounded the one-year anniversary of Mom's murder was completely absent for the second. There were no newspaper articles and no news stories to commemorate the anniversary. Even Candice, whom I spoke with fairly often, was busy with other commitments. Interest in Mom's case was dying, and my attempts to resuscitate it were fall-ing flat.

I still felt very strongly that nearly everything I encountered those days was a sign about Mom's case, so when I drove into the parking lot of my local grocery store early one Saturday morning and saw the small white SUV parked near the front of the lot with the words "1-800-AUTOPSY" in large print across the side, I had to stop. Pulling past the vehicle to find a space, I caught a small but meaningful detail. The image of a toe, with a toe tag reading,

"El Muerto,"—the dead one—was painted on the driver side door. That phrase resonated with me on so many levels. It spoke to the way I was personally feeling, totally numb, and the way the case felt to me—dead in the water. Sitting in my car, reading the list of services provided by the company that was conveniently printed in bullet point fashion on the back window, I couldn't shake the feeling that I needed to meet whomever owned that car.

No sooner had I had the thought than I saw a large tan skinned gentleman with a thick brown mustache exit the grocery store and head straight for the car. With my heart beating at an insane rate, that seemed to be its new norm, I took a breath and opened my door just as he approached.

"Hello," I said.

A huge, warm smile spread across his face, and he said, "Good morning."

"Good morning," I said, stepping closer and extending my hand, "I'm Lauri Taylor; do you have a minute?"

Extending his hand to me, he said, "Hello, Lauri Taylor, I'm Vidal Herrerra. How can I help you?"

With his kind invitation of help, I quickly blurted out two years of frustration, which he patiently soaked in. I then asked him the question I needed answered. "Do you know anything about Mexican autopsies?"

"Oh, yes, I do. What did you want to know?"

"Is it standard protocol during a Mexico autopsy to supplement the written document with autopsy photos?"

"Yes, it is. I've never seen one without."

"Thank you. You have no idea how helpful that information is to me."

With that, Mr. Herrera handed me his business card and told me to call him if I had any further questions. He jumped into his vehicle, probably headed towards his next autopsy. I stood in the parking lot for a moment staring at his card and knew precisely what my next move would be in Mom's case.

★   ★   ★

My obsessive tendencies and hyper focus around the case had paid off, and a little new life was breathed back into me. I was excited to phone Miguel Ortiz first thing Monday morning to ask, again, about autopsy photos. I had asked him so many times, it hardly seemed worth asking once more but, after speaking with Mr. Herrera, I just couldn't believe that authorities in San Felipe had not documented Mom's autopsy with pictures, so I tried to think of one more way to ask.

"Hola, Miguel, how are you?" I asked in my usual mixture of Spanish and English.

"Hola, Lauri, muy bien, gracias. Como estas?" he asked, in his usual happy-to-hear-from-you tone.

"Do you have time for a quick question?"

"Si, como no." *Yes, of course*, he answered.

"I have asked you about photos taken *of* my mother's autopsy many times, but I want to know if any photos were taken *before* her body was autopsied?"

Miguel paused for a minute, as though he were thinking and answered, "Si, si, yes, Lauri. There were photos taken before your mom's autopsy," he answered casually.

Oh holy cow, I thought. I was dumbfounded. I had been asking the wrong question the whole damn time. He thought I wanted to see pictures of my mother's corpse opened up like a frog in biology lab. Because I said "of" he had assumed I meant "*while* it was happening."

I thanked Miguel profusely for his help and hung up the phone, still a bit in shock. *They do exist, and I am going to get 'em. I thought.* I would have asked Miguel about getting the photos, but he had been moved about so much over the last year, his responsibilities were no longer in Ensenada where I would need his help. I had asked SDSO and Cal DOJ repeatedly for help getting the autopsy photos from Mexico with no response. I didn't want to betray my confidence with Miguel, so I would never tell anyone in the United States or Mexico where I had heard that the photos existed, but I would continue to pressure them all until we got them. I sat down at the computer and fired off several emails requesting the photos and the return of Mom's van, for good measure.

While I waited for responses to my emails, I decided to pour back through Mom's records. We had very limited financial information because the week after Mom disappeared, Adam's truck was broken into in Vista, and some of A&J's business records were stolen from the vehicle. I was curious about a short phone call Mom had received two days before she disappeared that I had tracked to Wells Fargo. I began to turn through the pages of the bank statement, and nothing was adding up.

For the last three months, Mom had barely been able to make the lease payment on the big store, and I couldn't imagine how she was paying for the small store, let alone her own living expenses. As far as I could tell, there would not have been enough money in her account to pay the lease on the big store on April 1. I had made it clear to Mom that my initial investment in her small consignment store was all that I was willing to give, because Rick and I had talked it through and that was what we agreed upon. Mom would have been forced to ask someone for money or figure out a quick way to make some cash.

Wringing my hands, as I contemplated the question of money, I looked down and examined them for a moment. My engagement ring and anniversary band glimmered in the sunlight that poured in through the kitchen window. I studied the face of my shiny designer watch, and the bands of the beautiful Tiffany ring I wore on my right hand, and they all began to feel like they were made of pure lead. They were suddenly heavy from the weight of the question I could not get out of my head: *Did Mom go to Mexico because of money? To make money selling drugs?* Flipping back through the stack of receipts and bank statements, I couldn't help but believe money was a likely motive and slowly slid my rings off my fingers and held them in the palm of my hand. I took the back off of my earring and slid it from my right ear, and did the same with the left, then rolled the small pile of diamond, gold and platinum jewelry in my palm and sobbed.

I had done the quick math, and what I held there in one hand could have easily paid Mom's lease on the new building. *Why didn't I just send her money?* The weight of my guilt about money was too heavy to wear every day like an anchor, so I placed everything except for my plain wedding band and my watch back in the velvet box they had come in, and I vowed not to put them back on until I proved that money was not the reason Mom had gone to Mexico.

★　　　★　　　★

Early in the summer of 2008, Candice returned from a long stretch of travel for work. I told her that I believed that it may be time to make an assessment in Mom's case, her best guess about what happened, and move on. Candice, as always, was supportive of anything I desired, but she reminded me that because I hadn't given up on asking about the autopsy photos, we knew that they existed. Her message was that my persistence usually paid off. The pep talk worked and I promised her and myself that I would refocus my efforts.

The signs about Mom's case continued to poke at me, in the oddest places. I took Clark and his friend Brian to the San Diego Sports Arena for a night out at the WWE One Night Stand wrestling event, which featured a "Last Man Standing" match between Randy Orton and Triple H. To be festive, I had worn a black wrestling t-shirt that Clark had given me with the words, "hustle, loyalty, respect," across the chest, and he and Brian had both laughed when they saw me in it. Walking out of the arena towards our car after the show, I looked across the parking lot and was surprised to see the friendly and familiar face of my cold case detective and his sons. Clark and Brian had already jumped in the car, when I stopped to speak to him.

"Hello, Tommy," I said, after hesitating for just a moment, worried about my credibility coming into question because of my fashion choice.

"Hello, Lauri," he said, containing his laughter and introduced me to his boys.

"Small world isn't it?" I laughed.

We chatted for a minute about the event, then parted ways, but not before I turned and yelled, "Call ya on Monday."

Tommy turned around laughing, "I'm sure you will, Lauri," which made me smile.

After my call with Miguel, I had revved back up on a full-scale email campaign, nearly reaching stalker status in the process, hounding every law enforcement and governmental agency for which I had a current mailing address. I was on a mission to recover the van and to acquire the autopsy photos from Mexico. To Tommy's credit, he took my often demanding correspondence in stride and, in fact, seemed to be working our case more than ever. He was starting to re-interview people in Vista, and was making a huge effort to connect with the investigators in Mexico. His effort and communication had reached a totally new level, and deserved recognition, so I emailed Ray Henry who, besides being Tommy's boss, was his close personal friend, to thank him for assigning Tommy to Mom's case.

At the same time SDSO seemed to be gearing up, Max Salazar who was the top dog at Cal DOJ, two ranks above Eduardo Reyes, stepped up as well. Max communicated directly with the commandante at the PGJE to request the return of the van and all reports, including the important autopsy report with photos. But over the summer months, the activity that had buzzed in June diminished quickly as it did every year when I backed off of the work on Mom's case to enjoy summer with Clark and Katy.

By September my sisters were all feeling frustrated that no progress was being made in Mom's case and, hoping to get some kind of closure, Kim suggested we go speak with a psychic. If nothing else, it sounded like it would be a fun and entertaining night out together. Kim, who is very well read, especially in true crime, researched psychics in the Los Angeles area who worked with law enforcement. She contacted Mikaela Green and set up an appointment. Sherri and Keith had already booked a vacation during that time, so Deb, Kim, and I went on our own. Kim emailed us the specific instructions that Mikaela had forwarded to her: drive together, be on time, and no perfume.

Mikaela's home was perched on a precarious but gorgeous hillside in Los Angeles. She opened the door to greet us, barefooted, in leggings and a tunic. She had the appearance of a former ballet dancer. Walking through her entry, I noticed a box of twisted silverware sitting on the polished hardwood floor. She saw me glance at it.

"It's called spoon bending. I do it psychokinetically, meaning with my mind," she said.

"Oh, that's amazing," I said, lamely. I had never heard of such a thing and wasn't sure what to make of it.

Mikaela led us to her living room, which was bordered on one side by stately bookcases lined with crystal balls of every size, shape, and color, and the latest works by Eckhart Tolle, which she also caught me spying. Kim, Deb, and I sat across from Mikaela, who had perched herself, cross-legged, in a cozy overstuffed armchair.

The only thing Kim had told Mikaela was that we were interested in information about our mother who had been murdered. Mikaela closed her eyes and began to speak, alternating between channeling a person and explaining what she was hearing. Right away, Mikaela felt as though she had connected with Mom, but she kept belching, which I found totally unnerving, and I shifted in my seat.

"Can she tell us what happened to her?" Kim asked.

"She doesn't want to talk about that right now," Mikaela said. "But she is happy to be here with her girls."

Hmmm, that's convenient, I thought to myself, pessimistically. Then Mikaela started to moan loudly, touching her head and her cheek, and then her knee and said, "She is showing me where it hurts."

Deb, Kim, and I sat mesmerized.

"The blood, the blood, the blood," she wailed, and the pessimist resurfaced in me. *She has no idea what she is talking about. There was no blood at the crime scene,* I thought, looking over at Kim whose expression screamed, "Ditto."

I continued to grow more uncomfortable sitting there, and Mikaela picked up on it and called me out.

"What's going on with you? Are you okay?" she asked.

"I'm fine, thank you," I fibbed.

Mikaela turned to Debbie, "There are books to be written, right?" she asked.

Deb looked at Kim and me, "Yes," she said.

"Two books, your mom said. A children's book, too."

The course of our reading then shifted off in bizarre directions, from Mikaela asking which one of us owned the French maid costume (to which we all pleaded innocent) to her channeling our grandfather's terrier mix, Skippy. Mikaela lost me for good when she recommended that I get healthy and "lose the weight." When the reading was over, I couldn't get out the door fast enough. Deb, Kim and I laughed hysterically, recalling the crazy evening over dinner and wine. At least we had a nice dinner.

★   ★   ★

As soon as I thought the case was winding down, it wound right back up again in November. Tommy, Max Salazar, and the PGJE had been communicating with me and each other. And to my complete amazement, it looked as though we were finally going to get Mom's van back. I coordinated a meeting at SDSO for early November, and for the first time in the case since Candice had joined forces with me, SDSO, Cal DOJ, my sisters, Candice, and I would have the opportunity to sit at the same table and discuss the next step in the investigation.

Deb, Sher, and Kim had never met Candice, so I arranged for all of us to have lunch together before we met at SDSO headquarters. They were thrilled to meet her, and she them. Candice wanted to explain why she felt it important to examine the van and have access to all reports and information regarding the case.

"In my job; I have to be open to all possibilities. I would be doing your family, and your mom a disservice if I did not question every possible scenario, and I need every bit of evidence we can get ahold of. When I met with Michael (Dr. Baden) last year, he implored me to do that, as well," she said. My sisters and I told Candice we were in agreement and would support her having access to all the evidence we could get from Mexico.

Tommy had reserved the conference room for us, and as we always did, my sisters and I took our seats together across from Max Salazar and a new Cal DOJ agent who was just introduced to us, named Armando Delgado, who were seated with Tommy, Ray Henry, and one other detective from SDSO. Candice sat with us. It very much felt like the boys against the girls, only at this meeting, the "boys" were on our side and ready to help.

Armando quickly explained that Cal DOJ had set up for the van and all the evidence in Mom's case to be shared with Candice and SDSO, but there was one hitch. Our family didn't have the registration to Mom's van, and even if we did, it would have been cost-prohibitive to pay the impound fee after two and a half years. Tommy offered a solution. If we didn't care about holding onto the vehicle, SDSO would provide a location for the van to be brought to the United States for examination, and would allow Candice and a forensic team from SDSO several hours to go over the van thoroughly. SDSO would process any evidence gathered, and the van would be returned to Mexico. I think even Candice was floored by the turn of events; my sisters and I certainly were. Tommy told us he would coordinate the date with Armando and communicate with me about Candice's availability. Armando concluded the meeting and asked if anyone had any additional questions.

"I do, thank you," I said to Armando, "Can I get your cell number?"

The entire "boy" side of the table broke into laughter. I was sure they were thinking, *Now its your turn to take all her phone calls.*

Tommy called me later that week to ask about Candice's schedule. I told him she would be in New York the first week of December for her annual trip, but the second week looked good.

"How does December 11th, look for you?" he asked.

I cleared the lump in my throat and answered, "It works for me."

Tommy didn't have a clue of the significance of the date that he chose. It was the anniversary of the last day I saw Mom, but I considered it a lucky omen—and maybe, my chance to clear my name and my conscience once and for all.

When my phone rang on Wednesday, December 9, I fully expected that Tommy was calling to firm up our plans for Friday, but that was not the case. He had bad news, really bad news. I hung up the phone and fell to a heap on the floor, crying. Later, after I had spoken to Candice and had composed myself, I typed out an email to my sisters:

December 9, 2008

Hi Sisters,

I have spoken with Tommy regarding the recovery of Mom's van this morning. We were supposed to be touching base to finalize plans to go to Calexico for inspection of the van on Thursday. Unfortunately, the news that I just received this morning is devastating . . . not only can Mexico not locate the remaining physical evidence in Mom's case (apparently they have moved offices), but now, they cannot locate the van either.

Armando from California DOJ followed up yesterday with officials in Mexico to basically say, "what the hell," and is awaiting their follow up in Mexicali. I will let you all know more info when I hear back from Tommy or Armando.

Love you,

Laur

It had been a long, disastrous year and I could not envision any way to proceed with Mom's investigation, given the latest development. Distraught and beaten, I wrote to Candice that I would be sending Christmas Cards with the inscription, "Merry Fucking Christmas!" With no additional evidence, there was nothing for Candice to do, or for Tommy to do, or for Armando to do, which meant that there would be absolutely nothing for me to do. This for me was "The Last Stand." I had lost the match by TKO, and it felt as though I had rightfully earned myself the stage name, "El Muerto." *The dead one.*

⊰⊱

SEVENTEEN

Lost and Found

The year ended on a very low note, with all the evidence in Mom's case including the van, lost somewhere in Mexico. At the holidays we made lame jokes about who might be driving Mom's vehicle around Baja, but despite the brief attempt at humor, the mood was pretty somber. With no physical evidence it would be difficult, if not impossible, to make a case, and the likelihood of a witness coming forward or someone confessing to the crime wasn't even worth a moment of thought.

The challenge for me now was to figure out the next step. We had been on a roll with Candice, SDSO, Cal DOJ, and the PGJE finally working together, cooperating and investigating. I could not have imagined this happening, even a year ago, but it was difficult to keep people interested and focused. Detectives, like the rest of us, are drawn to the things they believe they can be successful at, and the longer a case sits, the less likely it will be solved. My New Year's resolution for 2009 was to not lose hope for resolution in 2009.

Every year around the middle of March, very close to Katy's birthday, a large hedge in our yard (and yards all over Orange County) blooms with tiny pink flowers. When Katy was two, she sat in front of the hedge in a pale pink smocked dress for her birthday picture, and since then, when the yard becomes covered in pink, I know it is time to start planning my girl's birthday party. But now with the happy reminder of Katy's impending birthday, there also came the grim reminder of the ten days Mom was missing and the day that she died. Each year I believed it would get easier, but each year, I got sick, quiet, and reclusive for the days between March first and March twenty-fourth. There was no way around it. I hoped that someday the memory would not be so heavy and that the ribbon of guilt that tethered Katy's birthday with Mom's death would be undone, but that someday was not now.

Katy knew what she wanted for her 15th birthday. Like every other 15-year- old in the country, she wanted to see Taylor Swift's Fearless Concert Tour. Rick arranged to get tickets from the office so she could bring her closest friends who also loved T-Swift. Since the concert was not until May, I sat down at my computer to make up a cute IOU to put in Katy's birthday card. Unsure of the date of the concert, I went to the Staples Center website to confirm it before typing it on the page. The date listed for the concert was May 22, 2009. I sucked in my breath. There it was, again, the connection: Katy's birthday-gift concert would take place on Mom's birthday. No matter how I tried, I simply couldn't get away from Mom's story. I sat there and cried and cried as if the wound was brand new.

The three-year anniversary of Mom's murder, March 24, 2009, came and went without much fanfare: no newspaper articles, no television reports, and no meetings at SDSO. My sisters and I got together for dinner, and we talked about spreading Mom's ashes and we all agreed that we thought it would help us find closure. I said I would participate in anything they decided, because Mom's ashes didn't hold any great significance to me, but the real truth was, closure for me could only come when the case was closed. To reassure law enforcement that I was still on the case, I sent a slightly tart email to SDSO and Cal DOJ to remind them that it was the anniversary of Mom's death and that my family and I still expected answers. I sent the email even though I seriously doubted that finding answers, finding the truth, would be possible.

I had begun to believe that nothing I had hoped for would be possible.

Less than two weeks later, I was out in Palm Desert for a quick overnight during the kid's spring break from school. Clark was up early and out on the golf course for the morning. Katy and I were looking forward to time at the pool. I shoved my BlackBerry and my room key into my pool bag and we headed out.

We found our group. Katy and the girls jumped straight into the water while the moms made camp nearby the pool. The desert was an annual tradition for spring break and I felt truly relaxed among friends, knowing my kids were enjoying themselves, too. Just as I was sinking back into my lounge chair and sipping on a cool blended "vacation" drink with an umbrella, my phone blinged and I grabbed it. It was Tommy. I read his five-line email in a flash. *Omg, we are back in business,* I thought, nearly jumping out of my chair.

"What is it Laur?" my girlfriend asked, looking up from her magazine.

"I just got an email from Detective Nash. Armando, the agent from Cal DOJ called him today. They found some of the evidence from Mom's case and they are bringing it to San Diego next week."

"Cheers to good news," I said, lifting my cocktail towards the group for a toast. We all leaned in to clink our plastic cups, and I felt hopeful again for the first time in months.

I quickly replied to Tommy, thanking him for the update and asked him for Armando's cell number, explaining that I was on spring break and did not have access to my files. Tommy came through for me as always, giving me the phone number and told me to "Enjoy your time off." *Time off, not a chance*, I thought, stepping away from the noise of the pool to dial Armando.

For the second time that day, luck was on my side and he answered.

"Agent Delgado,"

"Hello, Armando, it's Lauri Taylor."

"Hello, Lauri, how are you?"

"I'm really well, thank you. I just heard from Detective Nash that you will be bringing the rope and the ball cap to San Diego."

"Yes, I have been pushing the Deputy DA about the recovery of the van and went through their evidence lockers when I met with them in Ensenada."

"Wow," I said, "I am speechless," feeling relieved and grateful for his initiative.

"That is what we are here for, Lauri. I have coordinated a meeting with SDSO, detective Velez, and the DA to review the work that has been done on your mom's case and hopefully to develop a joint strategy for moving forward in the investigation."

"I can't thank you enough. I had nearly given up hope of anything coming from Mexico. Can I ask you for one more thing?"

"Of course."

"Could you please check into autopsy photos, again? They are very important to me."

"Sure, I'll let you know."

After my call with Armando, I took Tommy's advice and tucked my phone away in my bag, rejoined my circle of friend's at the pool, and ordered another round of cocktails. I could breathe again, knowing there was movement in the case. Later that afternoon when I returned to my room, still buzzing with excitement about my call with Armando and from the affects of my poolside libations, I merrily emailed Candice and my sisters an update.

By the following week when my kids returned to school, I hadn't heard anything back from Candice, which was unusual. I was standing in the kitchen cooking dinner and noticed a Special Report news banner flash upon the screen with Candice's name and face along with it, and soon understood the reason for the delay. A few days earlier, in northern California, Melissa Huckaby had been arrested for the sexual assault and murder of a young child, Sandra Cantu. Huckaby, the mother of the preschooler's best friend, had stuffed her tiny victim's remains into a suitcase and tossed it into an irrigation pond.

The news anchor ran through Candice's resume: Ms. DeLong was the head profiler for the FBI in San Francisco, served as the liaison to the Bureau's world famous Behavioral Sciences Unit at Quantico, and was a member of the Child Abduction Task Force. I watched, in awe, as Candice coolly quoted statics about murder and sexual assault rates among female perpetrators. But I knew Candice; she would be furious and heartbroken about this little girl. Nearly every news channel and newspaper across the country featured Candice's opinion regarding the Cantu case. Two days later, coincidentally on the day that Mexican authorities were meeting with SDSO, I received an email from her apologizing for having not responded back to me right away. I told her, "No worries, I see you've been busy," and promised to call her if I heard anything from Tommy about the meeting.

Tommy called me while I was sitting in the parking lot of the high school waiting to pick up Katy on a Friday afternoon.

"I've got some good news for you today," he said proudly.

"I can't wait to hear it," I said, holding my breath and checking the clock to see how much time there was until Katy got out of school.

"Mexico handed over twenty-nine of your mother's autopsy photos yesterday. I guess Armando went to the PGJE and physically hunted down all the evidence himself."

"Oh my God," I said, "I can't believe it." I lay my head on the steering wheel, shocked, and began to cry quiet, happy, thankful tears.

Tommy, unaware that I was weeping, continued to brief me about the meeting.

"The quality of the autopsy photos is not up to US standards, but they are much better than I might have expected. We have taken the rope and the hat into evidence and will send them to the lab for analysis."

"Tommy, I want Candice to have those photos as soon as possible."

"Why?" he asked.

What the hell? I thought. Floored by his question, I shot up in my seat and wiped away my tears. The answer seemed so obvious to me, but I proceeded respectfully. "Because it is important for her to have access to all the evidence in the case so that she can make a determination of what happened to our mother for my family."

"Lauri, I understand, but we are trying to build a working relationship with Mexico and don't want to risk jeopardizing their trust by sharing the evidence they have just handed over to us," he explained. "Candice is not a forensic pathologist and I may want to send the photographs to one here in San Diego."

I hadn't even heard the school bell ring, but looked up and saw Katy approaching in the distance. *Now is not the time to argue this point*, I thought. "Okay, Tommy. I really appreciate all your time on this, thank you. I gotta run."

Katy jumped into the passenger seat next me and dropped her backpack on the floorboard. We were on our way to buy a dress for her to wear to the Taylor Swift concert, so I took off my investigator's hat for the moment, and we headed towards the mall. When Katy and I got home from shopping early that evening, she started on homework, and I sent Candice and my sisters the latest update. I should have been skipping for joy. The autopsy photos that we weren't even sure existed were now safely in the United States. I had lobbied HARD for those photos for three years and had helped to facilitate a relationship between SDSO and Mexico where only mutual mistrust had previously existed. I had asked Miguel Ortiz long ago to try to reopen the door with SDSO after he and the other detectives from Mexico felt betrayed and disrespected by Detective Long, and had rightfully convinced him that Ray Henry and Tommy Nash were the good guys. But as I recalled each point of my conversation with Tommy in writing, I became more and more outraged.

I'm calling Ray Henry first thing Monday morning, I thought. *I'm going to get those photos to Candice one way or another.*

The weekend passed slowly and would have been interminable had I not received a funny and encouraging email from Candice, restating her confidence in me and my ability to professionally handle my call with Ray Henry. The best part of the correspondence, though, was the news that Candice was coming to Los Angeles to film a segment for Dr. Phil, and she invited me to join her for dinner. It was always a treat to be with Candice, not only because we laughed so hard, but because we had become real friends and cared about one another's lives, children, and happiness. I felt like the best version of myself when I was with her because she never treated me like anything less. The phone call to Ray Henry was as much for her as it was for me and my family. Candice pushed me to get those photos, and she should have them.

★   ★   ★

As soon as the kids were off to school on Monday, I sat down with my coffee and dialed Ray Henry. Having the weekend to think about the call was probably a blessing, because it allowed me to think through my frustration. I owed Ray and Tommy my gratitude and respect, but I also owed it to myself to speak up. Speaking up still left me unsettled at times.

Ray picked up the line and greeted me with his usual kind and "happy to help you" attitude, and I got right to the point.

"I spoke with Tommy last week about sending the autopsy photos to Candice, and he told me that he would prefer not to send them to her because he didn't want to jeopardize the relationship with Mexico. Ray, you promised us that Candice could have access to all the evidence in Mom's case," I said, waiting and biting my tongue so I wouldn't fill the silence or let him off the hook.

I heard Ray heave a breath in, and he replied, "Yes, I did. I'll have Tommy copy them and send them out to Candice this week. Please email me her mailing address."

"Thank you, Ray," I said, "I really appreciate it." I hung up and had my moment of joy. *Yes!! This speaking up for yourself thing really works.*

It would be a few more weeks before Candice confirmed that she had received the package of photos from SDSO. She didn't have time to look at them right away because she was busy traveling for work. My anxiety was bubbling up every day because of the "hurry up and wait" nature of the last six months, but I tried to remain optimistic despite my impatience. I had hoped to be able to give my sisters some answers about the case before Mom's birthday, but it was not meant to be.

★   ★   ★

Friday, May 22, was a busy day in the Taylor household and the start to a hectic Memorial Day weekend. Rick, Clark and his good friend Austin got on the road early in the morning for a boy's trip to Las Vegas. They were excited to see the UFC 98 fight at the MGM Grand Hotel on Saturday night, which featured one of Clark's favorite MMA fighters, "Sugar" Rashad Evans. Katy and I had our own girls' weekend planned, starting with the long-awaited Taylor Swift concert that evening, and were out the door with friends by early afternoon so we could avoid the holiday traffic to Los Angeles.

Katy, her six girlfriends, my friend Karin, and I arrived at the Staples Center in plenty of time to catch the opening act, which was Kelli Pickler, a beautiful country artist who had gotten her start on American Idol. Taylor Swift put on an amazing show, and we all danced and sang and screamed and had a ball. During the final song of the set, I ran out to the ladies room and pulled my BlackBerry from my purse. I had three missed calls and a few texts from Rick. The noise was still very loud in the arena, so it was no wonder I hadn't heard my phone. I read through his texts first. Although they were vague—"I need to talk to you as soon as possible"—I knew something was very wrong. I just felt it.

Five minutes later, I had the whole story. Rick had experienced severe back pain at dinner and had blood in his urine. He was in too much pain to drive himself, and asked Clark and Austin to drop him at the hospital. In the ER they palpated Rick's abdomen, sent him for an MRI and found a mass on his kidney; from the size and appearance, they were nearly certain, without even doing a biopsy that it was cancer.

When I hung up, I could feel the blood had drained from my head. I remember thinking for a moment that I couldn't do it.

I couldn't handle another crisis, another emergency, another any-thing. But I had no choice. I walked back into the suite in a daze.

"Lauri, what is it?" Karin asked, searching my face.

"We have to get to Vegas," I said, and blurted out what I had learned.

Katy had planned a sleepover at our house for all the girls who came to the concert that night, but we needed to get to Las Vegas as quickly as possible. Rick was alone in the emergency room while Clark and Austin, two 17-year-olds, were alone at the hotel. I explained to Katy and her friends that Rick was in the hospital and we needed to reschedule the sleepover. They were all sweet and very concerned, and the hour drive home from the concert was agonizingly slow. I called my friends, Kelly and Tony, to ask for their help watching the dogs; Karin drove all the girls home for me; and I called Austin's mom, Pam, who was a new friend, to explain the odd situation. Katy and I packed a quick overnight bag and finally got on the road about 1:00 a.m.

We chatted for a while as we raced down the deserted highway, but Katy was exhausted and thankfully fell asleep, stretched out in the back seat, on her favorite comforter from home. When I was certain her eyes were closed, I called Clark and Austin, who were fairly unfazed considering they had just taken Rick to the ER in Las Vegas, a place neither of them had ever driven before. I called Rick next, and we could only speak briefly because his phone bat-tery was nearly dead, but I could hear the fear in his voice.

"You're going to be okay," I said, as if saying it would make it true.

For the next two hours, while Katy slept peacefully in her "Fearless" concert T-shirt, I drove and cried as hard as I have ever cried, filled to the brim with fear that just poured out of me, soak-ing the front of my own shirt and the thighs of my jeans. I could barely see the dark road ahead through my tears and considered pulling off to the shoulder, but I needed to get there, for Rick, for Clark, and for Katy, so I kept driving.

Why is this happening? I thought, *I can't do this. Is he going to die? He can't die —our poor kids have lost enough.* My thoughts were scrambled and unfocused, and my driving had become erratic, too, so I pulled off the highway to find a hotel. Katy sat with her blanket in an armchair near the front desk, while I checked us in.

"You're here just for the night?" the clerk asked.

"Yes, just for a few hours, actually," I answered.

"I'll need a credit card and a signature, ma'am."

The young man swiped my card and slid the registration slip across the counter, and handed me a pen. Struggling to focus, I searched the form for the signature line, and instead found myself staring at the check-in date: May 22, Mom's birthday. I opened my mouth to correct the error, because it was well past midnight, but the ribbon that tethered Katy's birthday, my mom and tragedy together, tightened around my throat like a noose, and I couldn't speak. *Am I still being punished?*

I managed to sign the form, Katy and I crashed as soon as we hit the room, and by 8:00 a.m. the next morning, we were in Las Vegas by Rick's side.

EIGHTEEN

Blood Run Cold

My phone did not ring about the investigation all summer because I had not placed a single call or written a single email to law enforcement, Candice, or the media, regarding the case. My family and I were busy riding the white-knuckle rollercoaster ride of Rick's kidney surgery and recovery. In June, however, I did receive a phone call on an entirely different topic that brought with it an additional gut check.

It was Deb. "Hey Laur, have you spoken to Kim?" she asked. I had seen that Kimi had left me a message, but I had been making a sandwich for Rick and hadn't had a chance to listen to the voice-mail yet. I knew immediately from Deb's tone, my intuition had sent a clear signal straight to my stomach, that something was wrong.

"No," I said.

Deb wasted no time in telling me the news. "Kim's mom is alive," she said.

The words hit me like I had been punched from behind and I stood up and began to pace. My heart filled with dread for Kim, and I felt nauseous, imagining her heartache and confusion over this shocking revelation. For forty-plus years we had all believed that Kim's real mother, Joan, had been unable to care for Kim and our brother Robbie, because of drug and alcohol abuse. We believed that Joan sent her kids to live with Dad and

223

Mom, and then at some point later, had taken her own life by drug overdose.

"Oh my God!" I said, "You have got to be kidding me! How can this be? Is Kimi, okay?"

"She's in shock," Deb said, "She kept repeating, 'Mom is alive, Mom is alive.' I thought she had lost it, Laur I thought she was talking about *Jane* until she told me about a phone call she had received."

Debbie quickly explained to me that Kim had gotten a phone message from a woman who claimed to be Kim's biological mother. This woman told her that she was dying and wanted to speak with her. When Kim couldn't reach me, she phoned Debbie to ask if she would follow up to find out if the story was true.

"It's her real mom, Joan Avila," Deb said.

"Why has it taken her this long to come looking for Kim?" I asked.

"Joan insisted that she had tried but said that Mom and Dad had forbidden her from ever seeing Kimi and Robbie."

I paced aimlessly, holding the phone to my ear, trying to remain as calm as I could, to take in this new information. Deb went on to explain that Joan was shocked to hear that Kim had believed she was dead for all these years and grief-stricken to hear that her only son, Robbie, a transient, diagnosed schizophrenic and drug addict, had died years before of complications from Type 1 diabetes and drug use. I became incredulous at my parents deceit. *Where the hell had the suicide story come from?*

Deb conferenced Kim into our call to discuss the unbelievable news, and each of us became increasingly incensed about having been lied to about Joan for our entire lives. Kim and I tried desperately to recall who had told us the story of her mother's passing, and when. Although neither of us could pinpoint an exact moment, Kim and I were fairly certain that Mom had told us during high school, at a time when our Dad was no longer living with us, and when Kim had become curious about her birth mother.

Debbie and I hung up with Kim and placed a call to our Dad to clarify the new information, but that call left us even more frustrated. Dad recalled being told of Joan's passing by a relative in their hometown, but had never heard the drug overdose version of the story himself. Dad told Deb and me that Joan had contacted him at work when she was destitute and incapable of raising the kids to ask him to take custody of them. Dad never recalled hearing from Joan after the day he picked up Kim and Rob to bring them to live as our new sister and brother in 1965.

Deb, Kim, and I talked later to rehash the upsetting news and tell Kim what we had learned from our call with Dad. We became convinced that Mom had created the drug overdose story to meet her own needs, to manipulate all of us into believing she was Saint Jane who had rescued Kim and Rob from a weak, selfish, and pitiful mother, and to keep Kim from knowing the truth. With Joan Avila dead, Mom knew that Kim would stop asking questions and not ever be inclined to search for the woman. Kim was robbed of ever having a positive thought or memory of her real mother.

The reality that Mom could develop and perpetuate such a vicious, cruel lie was sobering. For me, it cast a whole new light on the investigation of her death. Could I believe the evidence I was seeing? Could we believe anything about Mom? I needed answers, and I was going to get them for me and for my sisters as soon as things leveled off to some semblance of normal in my house.

That moment came in the fall. Clark started his senior year, and was busy filling out college applications; Katy began her sophomore

year, pushing through another round of golf tryouts in the August
heat; and Rick returned to work.

The first thing I did was email Tommy with a long list of very
direct questions regarding the autopsy photos and other evidence.
A week later, Sue and I had just finished a quick workout on
the hills in my neighborhood and stopped for an equally quick
lunch at our favorite taco joint, when my phone rang. Tommy
was returning my call, so I motioned to Sue that I would be just a
minute, and she grabbed the tray with our taco platters and took
it to a high table in the corner of the restaurant. I stepped outside
and paced about on the sidewalk while Tommy and I spoke on
the phone. When I returned to the tile-topped table, clutching my
BlackBerry, I sat down opposite Sue. She looked up at me from her
plate, a bit puzzled.

"Are you okay, Laur?" she asked, setting her fork down on the
plate.

"Blood," I said, leaning towards her, barely above a whisper.

"What, I didn't hear you?"

"Tommy says there was blood found on the rope from Mom's
van."

Sue's eyes opened widely and we both sat stunned for a minute.
She knew the significance of what I had just said, because I had
been sharing with Sue nearly everything about the case from
the start. The entire time, from that first day in Mexico when I
had scanned the report up and down in the little office of the
Minesterio Público hunting for the word "blood" in Spanish, to
the day that I had thoroughly examined all the photos taken by
Karla Nelson, I was looking for a single drop of blood. But there
had been no blood to be found—anywhere.

I pushed my tacos aside. Tommy had provided a lot of information to me on the call that I wanted to convey to my sisters and

Candice, as soon as possible. I sat and pounded out an email on my phone while Sue finished her lunch:

Hi Sisters,

Just wanted to give you a quick update on my conversation with Tommy. First, lab results have come back and they have found a female fingerprint/DNA on Mom's purse and would like to rule the sisters out as the source. We need to schedule a time to be swabbed, preferably next week, and he will meet us in the OC, if we would like. The rope was tested and came back with blood present. He did not say how much or where the blood was located. Finally, I had asked Tommy about the email address found on Mom's desk calendar (for the 47th time, poor guy) and he had an answer for me. The email address belongs to a couple from Washington State who was trying to have their mother's furniture consigned. The woman's name was "Lydia Alexander" as we had suspected and she and her husband do own a place in the Baja city of Mulege. He is an anesthesiologist. They told Tommy that they were simply potential customers and that they probably talked to Mom about a week before she went missing . . . interesting, but looks like maybe another big fat coincidence. Tommy didn't believe there was anything suspicious about their story and no further contact was required, but he is going to conduct some follow up interviews with Mom's acquaintances in Vista. Call me with any questions . . . and let me know if you have specific questions for Tommy so that I can ask them when I follow up with him tomorrow.

Love you all,

Laurs

We had hit another dead end with the email address, but I was encouraged by the work Tommy was doing on our behalf, and we were still eliminating potential suspects from the suspect pool—and that was progress. Tommy and I coordinated meeting times at my house for my sisters to have their DNA swabbed, but we had two small glitches in the scheduling. Sherri wasn't available at the same time as Kim and Deb, so Tommy and I arranged for her to come to my house the following week. The other issue was that my house had become a hospital ward with Clark and Katy suffering through a fresh outbreak of H1N1, the Swine Flu. I told Tommy not to worry because we could meet outside on the patio, and the doctor had given us the anti-viral medicine, Tamiflu. I found this fact to be another odd coincidence, because I didn't know what Tamiflu was until I had heard about Mom's obsession with the Avian Flu and her concern about a shortage of the drug. Between the time that Kim and Deb had come to the house and when Sherri was scheduled to arrive, I came down with the flu myself and was tired, achy, and impatient.

Sherri knocked and the dogs began to bark. I ran to the landing and through the small panes of glass at the top of my front door, I pointed towards the side gate and shouted, "Meet me in the back yard." We sat at the patio table just outside and I explained that I had a fever, the kids were sick inside, and I didn't want to risk Sher catching a nasty flu. My head pounded but I needed to run something past her before Tommy arrived.

"Sher, I am completely over this investigation and I am tired of tippy toeing around SDSO. What do you think about us just straight out asking Tommy about the blood?"

"Let's do it. What is the worst thing that can happen?"

"I don't know because I am feverish and can't think straight," I laughed.

Tommy arrived and gave Sherri the DNA swab kit, and instructed her to wipe the large Q-tip along the inside of her cheek, then insert the cotton end into a plastic container to be sealed and placed in a small manila envelope. Tommy sat at the head of the table with Sherri and me seated in patio chairs on his left and right. After Sher had completed her test, she handed Tommy the envelope and while he placed it in his briefcase, she gave me bug eyes from across the table, cocked her head and raised her Brooke Shields-like eyebrows at me. I gave her a tiny, knowing nod of acknowledgement and turned to ask Tommy a question about the blood.

"Tommy," I said, "Last week you mentioned that there was blood found on the rope. Was there any other blood found?"

"Yes, there was blood found on the blue ball cap, and there was a significant amount of blood in the van," Tommy said.

Significant amount of blood?

"What do you mean by significant?" Sherri asked.

"It's in the pictures from Mexico," Tommy said, incredulously, looking at Sher and then at me.

"We haven't seen the pictures from Mexico and Candice has not seen any pictures with blood in them," I said, "Can you show us . . . please?"

I knew how Tommy felt about protecting the evidence, but he reached into his briefcase, anyway, pulled out a big, thick binder and placed it on the patio table. He opened the pages slightly, rifling through them quickly, then split the notebook wide open, flashing the picture at us, then slammed it shut. That was all he was going to give us, and even though I only caught a quick glimpse of the photo, I could see very clearly that Tommy was not exaggerating about the amount of blood. The carpet in the back of the van was a light grey color, and because the seats were removed, the carpeting was unobstructed in the picture. Not just a few drops of blood, but a deep, red wine colored mass stretched across the picture.

"Candice doesn't have this photo. Can you send it to her?" I asked.

"She should have it. I sent it with the rest."

"I promise she does not have this one, Tommy."

"Okay, I will send it."

"One more thing," I said, "we talked last week about you sending the copy of the border-crossing video to Naval Intelligence to take a look for us. Any chance you can get that done?"

"I'll see what I can do, Lauri," he said.

And that was it. Tommy packed up his briefcase and I walked Sherri and him to their cars parked out front. Walking back to the house, I could feel my fever starting to spike, cheeks hot and head throbbing. I began to shiver. *That was a lot of blood . . . my Mom's blood. Oh my God, the psychic was RIGHT.*

★   ★   ★

I spent the next two days in bed, and on the third day got up to try to eat something. When Katy came in from school, she yelled to me in the kitchen, from the front door.

"Hey, Mom, there's a package here for you on the front porch," she said.

"Thanks, sweetie," I yelled back, "Just leave it on the front table for me."

I tried to keep my tone casual, but I was cringing inside, hoping Katy didn't hear the worry in my voice, and happy she did not know the contents of the package that Candice had sent to me overnight. It was a copy of all the autopsy photos that I had waited so long to get into Candice's hands, and even longer to see myself. Candice had copied each of the horrific photos for me, and they were stacked in that package, sitting on my front table in the same place where the bills and catalogs usually sat.

Candice had her own set of photos, plus two additional ones: the photos of the blood from the interior of Mom's van. Tommy had gone on vacation right after he'd left my house and had been unable to send the copies, so I had called Ray Henry to ask if he could fax the van photos to Candice. He didn't hesitate, and so now Candice had a complete set.

"Okay, love you. I'll be back around six," Katy said, slamming the door behind her.

"Love you," I yelled just as the door clicked shut. I ran to the entryway to retrieve the red, white, and blue cardboard envelope resting on the glass-topped console table. I scooped it up in both hands and stared at the packing label for a long time. *From Candice DeLong*, it read. The package was thicker and heavier than I imagined it would be, as though it contained a manuscript. *I have waited three and a half years for this moment*, I thought.

Months before I hired Candice, and before I could confirm that photos were taken during Mexican autopsies, I had lobbied San Diego Sheriff's Office, Cal DOJ, and the PGJE to get the pictures inside this envelope, and after Miguel Ortiz divulged to me that the photos actually existed in evidence, I became nearly obsessive with email requests for them. That package came about as a result of the relationships I had developed and was the culmination of a lot of hard work and determination, evidence that my family or I would never have seen, had I simply given up or stopped asking questions. But this reality did not make it any easier for me to open the envelope. I hoped that I was finally holding the key to the investigation in my hands, but I didn't want to see it, because the truth lay somewhere in a stack of photos of my mother's corpse.

Although I considered myself a decent detective, I never got used to seeing Mom's dead body. I had seen plenty of pictures—more than a daughter should—and I couldn't stop now. My chest felt heavy, everything felt heavy. I reminded myself to breathe, and stepped down the two stairs to the upholstered bench that flanked one end of our living room, placing the envelope squarely in my lap as I sat down. Running my hand over the top of the package, I grabbed the pull-tab and zipped the envelope open with one swift tug, throwing the long strip of cardboard on the seat cushion beside me, then pulled the stack of paper from inside. Just as I was about to set it in my lap, the hum of the garage door rolling up startled me to my feet, and I scrambled to cram the pictures back into the envelope. Heart racing, I ran to hide the package in a cabinet in the laundry room, and the back door flew open.

"Hey, Mama," Clark hollered, unaware that I was just a few steps from him.

"Hey, Clark," I said, quietly, trying not to startle him.

"Oh, wow," he said, jumping back. "I didn't know you were right there. What have you been up to?"

"Nothing much, Sweetie," I said smiling, my heart thumping so hard I could feel it in my throat. "How was your day?"

Clark's interruption had given me a reprieve from facing the stack of autopsy photos I had hidden in the cabinet, but it had reminded me of what else I was hiding. My obsession with Mom's case was making me sick with anxiety, and try as I might to balance it all out with therapy and exercise, I was losing the battle. Often, people would ask me, "How can you do this, it's your mother?" I would brush them off, saying, "You would do the same for your mother," but I was fairly certain that not everyone would. I never told anyone that I was driven by vicious, nagging, survivor guilt that gave me raging anxiety and sleepless nights. I was completely worn out by the investigation and by the charade.

I left the photos in the cabinet while Clark was in the house, which meant they were there all afternoon and evening. Candice texted me around 5:00 p.m. to confirm that I had received the package. We made a plan to go through the pictures together the following morning when the kids were in school. As soon as the coast was clear, Clark and Katy sitting safely in their first period classes, I went to the laundry room, Bailey and Bella at my heels, to grab the package. I sat down at my investigative workspace, the kitchen table, and dialed Candice.

"You ready, Laur?" she asked

"As ready as I'll ever be," I said, pulling the stack of photocopied pictures from the sleeve.

"Let's go through and number them, so we can reference them later, "Candice said.

"Okay, I'm ready," I said, staring down at the image of Mom's rigid, bruised, lifeless body, laid out on a silvery stainless steel table, her mouth agape, as though she was trying to say something to me. And wished I could say something to her, like exactly how much I missed her.

When Candice and I concluded going through the stack of autopsy images and the two images from the interior of Mom's van, which did show a significant amount of blood, she had made up her mind about what needed to happen next.

"I want to take these photos and the interior shots of the van back to Michael next month. Okay?" She was talking again about Dr. Baden. She was talking about the fact that there was so much more now to the story.

"Yes, whatever you think," I said, because my brain could not.

NINETEEN

❧❧

All Alone with My Memory

In early December 2009, Candice took the autopsy photos and all the evidence we had in Mom's case back to Dr. Baden in New York for analysis. It was time to get to the bottom of what happened to my mom, and Candice believed that we finally had enough evidence to make a determination, albeit a circumstantial one. I had booked and confirmed Candice's hotel room for the following week, although Candice had not yet heard back from Dr. Baden as to his availability for a meeting. She was confident he would phone back and make time to see her while she was in New York.

At that point, I wasn't confident about anything, and felt as though this opportunity with Candice and Dr. Baden was truly the last shot. If something conclusive didn't come from Candice's meeting with Dr. Baden, I would have trouble justifying spending any more money or time on the case. An inconclusive end could be near, and even though I promised Candice I would be open to any conclusion she arrived at, I couldn't stand the thought of not finding the truth.

Candice knew me well and sensed that I was uptight about the uncertainty of the trip (the barrage of texts I sent may have tipped her off) and she used her humor to diffuse my anxiety. On Tuesday, December 8, Candice flew to New York and wrote that she had to stop texting with me because Tiger Woods, who was in the middle of a marital scandal that had been splashed across the headlines, was "waiting for her next text." Then, cheerfully, she instructed me to "have a glass of vino and chill," which was sage advice considering my state of mind, so I did.

The following morning, true to her word and elated that she had come through for me, Candice texted me to confirm that she had spoken with Dr. Baden and planned to meet with him and his wife for dinner on Friday, December 11, 2009. That date would mark four years to the day since Mom and her girls sat in a theatre at the old Aviation High School, enjoying the music and watching the story of Grizabella and the cast of *Cats* on stage. It was the last time I saw or touched or spoke with my mother, and the years were causing her to fade from my memory. I could no longer hear her voice in my head, and too often, the only image I could conjure was of her contorted face from the stack of autopsy photos that were etched in my memory.

Early evening on Friday, my phone rang and my heart skipped for a moment when I pulled it from my pocket and read, "Candice DeLong" on the caller ID.

"Hey, how are you?" I asked, grabbing a notebook and pen from my nightstand.

"I'm good, thanks. Are you in a place where you can talk?"

"Yes, I am," I said, my hand shaking as I pulled the bedroom door closed behind me, and walked over to the chenille armchair next to the window to sit down.

"I'm very sorry to have to tell you this, Lauri," she began, and my mind raced to try to figure out what news could be bad. At this point, what news could possibly warrant that opening? ". . . but Dr. Baden and I agree that your mom was not murdered."

Not murdered? We'd been searching for a someone for four years. I had put everything else aside in my life to search for a murderer. What was she saying?

"That wound on her left wrist appears to be a classic self inflicted injury," Candice explained, "Your mother was right handed, correct?" her voice trailing off for a moment.

I sat, still and silent, staring at the black spiral bound notebook I had placed on the ottoman in front of me. I picked up my pen and leaned over to write, the tears rolling wildly down my cheeks. I spelled out the word in all caps—S-U-I-C-I-D-E—the ink on the paper smearing as I wrote each letter on the damp paper. Suicide. My mother had slit her own wrist.

"Lauri, are you there? Are you okay?" Candice asked.

"I'm fine, I'm fine . . . Go ahead, I'm listening." I said, wiping my chin on the sleeve of my sweater, numbed by the sight and sound of the word I had just written and repeated in my head.

Candice gently continued to recount her conversation with Dr. Baden, explaining that Mom had not actually bled to death from her slashed wrist. The blood loss from Mom's wrist injury was not an arterial bleed, which would have caused her to bleed out and die in a very short period of time, but was a substantial enough loss, maybe a quarter of her total blood volume, to cause her body to go into shock.

When the body is in shock it becomes susceptible to hypothermia (the reason accident victims are covered with a blanket). In the initial stage of hypothermia a person will shiver; this is the body's attempt to try to generate heat through the muscles. And then comes a phase called the "umbles," where a person may stumble, mumble, fumble, and/or grumble. At this stage, because of confused thinking and lack of motor coordination, a person is not fully aware that he or she needs help or medical assistance and may fall repeatedly, as if intoxicated, which explained the bruises and marks that made it appear as if Mom was beaten.

As hypothermia gradually progresses and the body begins to tire, there can be a sudden surge of blood to the limbs that can make victims feel as though their skin is burning. The deeply hypothermic victims will rip the clothes from their own body, exacerbating their condition by removing the body's last layer of protection, hastening unconsciousness and death.

"Your mom didn't know she was dying, Lauri."

"She undressed herself?" I pleaded.

"Yes, the phenomenon is called 'paradoxical undressing.' It is a paradox because the victims are freezing to death but take off their clothes because of the feeling of intense heat from the sudden rush of blood to the extremities."

I took copious notes, scribbling down every detail of Dr. Baden's explanation for his findings in Mom's death, but it was simply a robotic effort. My mind was unable to process it all because my thoughts were elsewhere. *How do I explain this to my sisters or to my children, or to Adam, who may unnecessarily feel the burden and weight of this information?*

"Dr. Baden asked about any history of mental illness," Candice said.

I cringed and thought, *borderline personality disorder?* Probably. Likely. Quite possibly. Months ago, after giving a detailed description of my turbulent and unpredictable upbringing to my therapist, she had suggested the diagnosis of Borderline Personality Disorder for Mom. The therapist became quite a bit more convinced of the diagnosis, after she had spoken with my sisters, that the life we had viewed as "normal" was, indeed, not, by therapeutic standards. It was simply "our normal." She asked if anyone in law enforcement had ever inquired about my mother's mental health. And no one had. "Why, Candice?" I managed to ask.

"Some diagnoses have a higher rate of suicide attached to them," Candice explained, "and BPD is one of them."

I tried desperately to stay engaged in our conversation and continued to write every word that Candice said to me, but lost my ability to concentrate on anything but the words "Suicide" and "Mental Illness" which I had written, repeatedly, down the page. I'm not sure I even thanked Candice when we finally got off the phone, but I needed time to just sit with the information by myself. Despite my partnership with Candice and my closeness with my sisters, I had felt alone throughout much of the investigation of Mom's death, but never more alone than in that moment in my chair. Suicide? *How could she do this to us?*

Over the last four years I had faced down many fears, but none as big as the one I was staring at now: the truth. And it was nearly unbearable because I was completely responsible for it. Because of me, because I couldn't let it go, because I needed to prove that I was not to blame, because I was suffocating in guilt and shame, my family would be saddled with this answer forever. *Debbie, Sherri, and Kim will feel guilty, Adam will feel guilty, and I will never be free of my guilt because I didn't do everything within my power to save Mom from this fate.*

Was this life's cruelest lesson or most profound? I had frantically searched for the truth, but it wasn't *the* truth that I wanted. I wanted to be free of the burden of responsibility, and now I would carry it with me like Jacob Marley's chain, for eternity. I seethed with anger at myself. After all that effort to make my mom, my sisters, and my entire family proud of me, I would instead be serving up a fresh course of heartache for the family to feast on at the holidays. I couldn't stand the thought of telling my family, ever, let alone at Christmastime. They had been through enough. I decided to wait until the new year to tell them. That would also give me additional time to prepare fully to deliver the verdict: guilty.

While Clark and Katy were in school for the last few weeks before their winter break, I poured over my notes from my conversation with Candice. From time to time, one of them would catch me crying and I would explain away my tears, which they

had gotten used to during my work on the investigation. I painstakingly researched the information that Candice had given me
about shock, hypothermia, and paradoxical undressing so that I
could explain them with confidence to my sisters. I also delved
into the topic of borderline personality disorder, hoping to make
some sense of this revelation about my mom.

★   ★   ★

In the weeks before Christmas, I found comfort and validation
in the words of Christine Ann Lawson's book, *Understanding the
Borderline Mother*. I loved my mom dearly and desperately wanted
to understand her. I knew in my heart that although Mom's mental
health had often prevented her from doing what was best for me,
her soul wanted what was best for me. She had given me many
valuable gifts, including a positive attitude, resourcefulness, and the
desire to make the most of my life. Mom had done the best that
she could in raising me, and in the moments that she was fully
present, she was larger than life. Her words were magic to me,
and because of her I believed I could do or be anything I imagined—even become a part-time homicide detective. My sisters and
I would giggle, though, when Mom would say, "I must have done
something right raising you girls," because she never understood
that this statement epitomized our relationship. Our successes were
hers, never our own.

Mom once shared with me how much she loved the poem
"Children Learn What They Live." I loved that poem, too, but the
reality in our family was that because of my mother's psychiatric
disorder, we had all learned some tough lessons. The unpredictability of my central caregiver, and the gap between her perception
of reality and my perceptions left me an anxious, frightened child
with pervasive self-doubt. I felt completely responsible for my

mother's happiness, doing everything I could to win her approval, to make her proud and to make sure she never got upset. I lived as a human mirror, a reflection of the person my mother needed me to be, because at her core she lacked her own sense of self.

If I dared to assert my opinion or take the other side of an argument, I was punished, vilified, and banished for my disloyalty. My worth was determined by my ability to meet her needs. This behavior set me on a path of people-pleasing, which in turn caused me to put a higher value on the feelings of others than on my own. I had indeed learned what I lived.

★   ★   ★

My "aha" moment about my relationship with Mom came when I finally realized that nothing I could have done would have been enough for her. Nothing. No amount of love, money, attention, or undying loyalty could have saved Mom, because she created and lived her own reality. Her reality was clouded by her illness, a condition the experts call "perceptional distortion." What could possibly have saved my mom was someone knowing that she lived with BPD and encouraging and assisting her to get proper care. My crime was not having any idea that something was truly wrong. I had grieved the death of my mother, had learned to use my voice to ask for the help I needed to find the answers I had to know, but still wrestled with the twin beasts that were my shame and guilt. What would I do if my family could not forgive me for finding this awful truth? A truth I never intended to find.

★   ★   ★

The first week of January, I asked Sherri if we could get together at her house so that I could tell everyone about Candice's trip to visit Dr. Baden in New York. They were all aware that she was going to see Dr. Baden, but I had brushed my sisters off before Christmas, fibbing that Candice hadn't had time to get back to me. After dinner I ran out to my car to grab the stack of notebooks that I had prepared over the holiday, a little surprised that no one had tried to discuss anything with me while they were eating. I hadn't eaten a bite. Adam, Tiffany, and Keith stayed downstairs and watched TV, while Deb, Sher, Kim, and I went upstairs to the privacy of Sherri's home office.

Handing each of my sisters a notebook, I took a deep breath and steadied myself to deliver the news. I asked them not to open their binders until I was done with my explanation. They would have the material to refer to later, if they needed it. I reviewed, point by point, the information that Candice had conveyed to me: the slashed left wrist, the large amount of blood in the van, shock, hypothermia, paradoxical undressing, and suicide. And I told them about Mom's probable diagnosis of borderline personality disorder.

The look on their faces was almost more than I could take. All three were staring at me with eyes that were wide, blank and expressionless. I recognized the look—it was disbelief. It was the same look that had greeted me every morning when I looked in the mirror for the past three weeks. I knew that there was a question screeching in their heads, tormenting them. It was like trying to shush a crow, though; the more you begged it to stop, the louder it got: *How could she do this to us?*

The air had been totally sucked out of the room. Deb glanced down at the notebook on her lap, picked it up with both hands, and looked back at me.

"So Mom really did this?" she said, her hands tightening around the binder.

I simply nodded back. For the better part of four years, every law enforcement organization involved in Mom's case insisted that she had been murdered and we believed them. As it turned out, they were wrong. Very wrong. What was there to say in the face of that fact?

Sher was consumed in thought, and Kim was not ready to accept suicide as the answer and told me so. I understood her feelings. There were still a lot of unanswered questions about the case: where was Mom for ten days, who was she with, why did she go to Mexico, and why did she go way out to that godforsaken stretch of desert by the sea? The case we had was circumstantial, but it was the only theory in nearly four years that completely added up. It had taken me every bit of three weeks to digest all the information I had just given them, and I still could barely believe it. I wondered how long it would take my sisters to fully accept the scary truth I had just clobbered them with.

Why was this new information so difficult for all of us to accept? Why was it easier to deal with a murder than a suicide? If I had found a murderer, there would not have been a beautiful party thrown or a parade through town, but there would have been a trial, a judge, a jury, and someone else to blame. The shadow criminal we had each carried with us would have had a face and a name. When everyone believed Mom had been murdered, my sisters and I were clearly victims deserving of sympathy and compassion. Now it felt as though we were accomplices, sentenced to carry our rightful share of shame and blame for the crime our mother had committed against herself.

The questions poured from all of us. How do we tell everyone? Who do we tell and when? It wasn't like we could send out a press release: "No Murderer Found—Jane Takes Her Own Life." Although my sisters did not speak it, I recognized their shame and embarrassment about having to share that Mom was not murdered, because I felt it, too. It was apparent to me that more time was needed to process the latest blow. We all agreed that we would share the new information with those whom we felt comfortable telling, in our own time, in our own way. Sherri and I discussed telling Adam, Tiffany, and Keith, and she was concerned about getting the explanation right. I asked if she would like for me to tell them for her, and she said she would. Deb and Kim stayed together in the office for bit, while Sher and I went downstairs to explain our findings.

Following Sher down the steep wooden stairs from her office to the family room below, where Adam, Tiffany, and Keith were watching television, I drew in a deep breath and gripped the rail. I was only partially done delivering devastating news, and I worried the most about telling Adam the truth about his beloved grandmother. Despite the fact that he had quit working with her the week before she disappeared, he guarded her memory fiercely and would not engage in any conversation about her that was less than complimentary.

With the three of them huddled in a semi circle of chairs in front of me, and Sher beside me, I replicated the speech I had just delivered to my sisters. Tiffany shrieked and cried, "How could she do this?" Keith was deeply saddened, pulling his black-framed glasses from his face to wipe his tears. "She must have been in so much pain," he said out loud, to no one in particular.

Adam took the news hard, as well, but in addition to his sadness, I saw something else—a bit of relief in his eyes. The nightmare of not knowing and constantly speculating about what happened to Mom could stop now.

"It's finally over," Adam said.

"It is sweetie," I said, tears spilling down my face.

"We don't have to think about this every holiday, every birthday, anymore," he said, looking at his feet, shaking his head in disbelief. After a moment, he lifted his head to look at me and said, "Without your tenacity Auntie Lauri, we would never have gotten an answer."

I ran to him, and jumped up to throw my arms around his 6′5″ frame, hugging and crying, so relieved that no one, especially Adam, resented me for having found the truth. After a minute, he pulled away from me, took a step back, and asked, "Have you ever considered doing this for a living?"

I let out a gasp, and we all busted out laughing.

"No, I mean it!" he said.

His question seemed ludicrous, but it reminded me that this wasn't quite over yet. I still had to make a trip to SDSO to close the case for good.

TWENTY

Case Closed II

All that remained for us to do was to officially close the case with the San Diego Sheriff's office—which brought me smack up against the fantasy I'd held in my head all these years as I'd fought to find the truth. There was no killer—which meant there would not be a shining movie moment for me. I would not be held up as the clever, resourceful golden child/crime solver. There would be no big headlines in the newspaper, no crowning moment of absolution. My vivid imagination, which had spun that fairy tale ending, actually foretold some of the important details of my feature film, like solving the case and returning to SDSO with key evidence.

But late in the third act, because I had not and could never have imagined the truth, the real truth, my story held a surprise ending. It was a vicious twist, for both my family and me. While I believed I was hunting a murderer, what I had relentlessly stalked for all those years was someone to blame for Mom's death—other than myself.

Finding a guilty murderer, most assuredly, would not have brought us any joy, but it might have cleared a guilty daughter of all self-imposed charges. Although I did not feel triumphant or proud about solving the case, I was comforted by the fact that against all the odds my family now had the closure they deserved. It wasn't the end that my brain had written, but it was good enough. I had a strong desire to finish what I had started, the right way, and that included a trip to SDSO to hand them the evidence necessary to close the investigation of my mother's murder for good. There were many blessings for us throughout the investigation, and having Sergeant Henry and Detective Nash in our corner was one of them. Their willingness to work with me and with Candice had been a big turning point in the case. Ray and Tommy deserved to know the truth.

When Debbie and I went down to the station together that day, and took our seats at the huge homicide conference table where we had held many meetings over the years, we first thanked Ray and Tommy for their hard work. Then with my black notebook in front of me for comfort and reassurance, I made my speech about the findings—what Candice and Dr. Baden had found about Mom's left wrist injury, what they believed the significant amount of blood meant, the fact that suicide was the only answer that completely made sense, and the diagnosis of borderline personality disorder.

I will always feel humbled and thankful when I remember Ray's incredible praise: *"Never in my more than twenty-five years of experience have I ever had someone from the outside come in and contribute anything to a case, let alone solve the case, which I fully believe you and Candice have done. You should be incredibly proud of yourself."* And when he added that my mother would have been proud of me, too, I swallowed the lump that swelled in my throat and held back my tears.

We had wrapped up our discussion, and as the four of us lapsed into casual chitchat, I found myself reluctant to get up from the table and leave the room. One last question still haunted me. Ever since Dr. Baden and Candice's presentation of the facts, a nagging thought had wormed its way into my head: where was the weapon? If my mother had indeed slashed her wrist, what had she used to do it? We would never know why my mother had gone to Mexico, or what had driven her to her final, violent act, but knowing about that one last piece of evidence would be a comfort to me—in a strange way, a confirmation of all that we had learned.

That was when I asked Tommy about the lack of a weapon and when he kindly offered to look over the photographs one more time. When he got up to get the file, Ray, Debbie, and I sat there, expecting nothing. My question had been a formality. Tommy knew that, Sergeant Henry knew it. We had gone over those photos time and time again, and Tommy was really just being nice.

When he came back to the table, sat down, and began to flip through the pictures, he then made his stunning three-word declaration—"There it is."

He tossed the photo towards me and I watched it hang in the air and glide into place right in front of me.

"Oh, fuck," I screamed, "Oh fuck!"

There, lying on the floor mat in the front seat of Mom's van was a large black knife. It looked like the kind of knife I imagined a hunter might use, thick handled with a curve at the tip of the blade.

I could not hold back my tears anymore. The image of that big knife clutched in my mother's hand was simply too overwhelming. She was the fugitive I had been hunting all along. She had committed this terrible deed. The truth that stared back at me from that picture was suddenly too much to bear. My chin dropped to my chest and I squeezed my eyes closed to try to shut it out, then pushed the picture away in Debbie's direction, and heard her let out a low gasp.

It had been such a difficult and harrowing puzzle to solve, and against all the odds, at long last, we had the final missing piece.

TWENTY-ONE

Death of a Stray

"Hey, Clark, let's go! Everyone is waiting for us at Don Gustavo's," I yelled towards his room.

"Sorry Mama, I'm coming," he yelled over the railing, bolting down the stairs.

"I had to grab a sweatshirt; it just started raining."

Realizing he was right about the weather, I grabbed my jacket on the way out the door, and ran with it covering my head, jumping in behind the wheel as quickly as possible to avoid getting soaked. Clark had already started the car and was adjusting the radio, when I touched my stomach and felt it rumble.

"Seriously, Clark, do you not feel that?" Thump, thump, thump, the windows rattled to the beat.

"Mom, you cannot possibly listen to rap without the base on the highest setting."

"Oh, I can and I do! Please turn it down. I feel sea sick."

With a grudging smirk on his face, he turned the dial back a tiny bit and we both laughed, as I pulled out of the driveway, Notorious B.I.G. blaring in our ears.

Pulling around the corner, I could see traffic starting to back up on the slick road ahead. As we approached the signal, Clark and I exchanged puzzled looks. "Did you hear that?" I asked, not sure what I had heard because the music was turned up so high.

Just as Clark opened his mouth to respond to me, a loud, piercing, agonizing wail suddenly drowned out the music. We both scanned the scene for the source of the cries.

"Oh my god, Clark, that dog has been hit."

We watched for a moment, in stunned disbelief, as the signal turned green, and all the cars pulled wildly in every direction to get around the writhing animal. I slammed my car to the curb just short of the intersection and threw the parking brake on while cars impatiently honked their horns and pulled around me.

"Stay here, in case you have to move the car," I said, and jumped out, unsure of what I was going to do next. Just as I stepped a foot on the curb, I looked up and saw a small white Mercedes slam to a stop, inches short of hitting the poor struggling dog, again. The dog's first assailant had apparently already fled from the scene, escaping in the mass exodus. A large bearded man exploded from the Mercedes, clearly agitated by the inconvenience of the stop. He grabbed the distraught, crying animal by its hind leg and dragged it to the gutter in front of me. I turned and ran, tears streaming down my face, back to the car where Clark was waiting for me.

"Is he going to be okay, Mama?" he asked.

"I don't think so, Sweetie, I can't leave him." I breathlessly dialed Animal Control, giving them the pertinent information about the dog's injuries, my desire to get him to a vet as soon as possible, and our location.

"Clark, text Dad and tell him to swing by and pick you up."

He did as I asked.

I really didn't want for Clark to have to see the injured dog. We'd had enough death in our home over the last four years. I drove around the corner, just past where the accident had occurred and parked so that my windshield would be facing away from where the dog lay crying and floundering. Rick arrived quickly pulling up right next to us and Clark gladly hopped in with him.

Walking back up the hill, I approached the pup slowly. He cried out and I jumped back. The street was dark and completely empty now, except for two cars that had had a fender bender trying to avoid the thrashing dog. Ten yards away, the two men, whose vehicles appeared unscathed, stood arguing in the street, oblivious to the creature whimpering on the asphalt.

"Shhhh, boy, it's okay," I called to the dog, afraid to get too close because he was in so much pain, but moved closer anyway. I watched his broad, smooth chest rise and fall, thankful to see him still breathing. I could hardly breathe myself. I had never witnessed a living thing, save for a few goldfish in my childhood, actually die, but I knew as I stood there in the rain that death was this dog's fate.

"It's alright boy, close your eyes."

It had been four years since Mom died, and even though I knew vaguely, scientifically, how she died, my nightmares did not stop. My brain worked overtime to fill in the blanks that were left unanswered by my investigations. The old dream was replaced with a new modified version, equally as violent and perhaps more disturbing than the previous one. Instead of the anonymous face of a killer, I could see my mother's face, and it was too much to bear, knowing what she was about to do. I could hear myself saying, "*Close your eyes*," but I was dreaming; they *were* closed, and the images kept coming.

Even more disconcerting than the images, was the dialogue that played in my head. What was she thinking at that moment when she grabbed the knife, slicing into the thin flesh of her wrist, blood pouring out and soaking the carpet of the van, while she waited to die? Did she choose to do this on Katy's birthday to punish me, to make a point that I was not there for her? Or was it something else?

Standing under the street lamp, I knelt down to get a closer look at the poor shivering pup. Or was I the one shivering? He lifted his nose slightly, trying to get a look at me, then let out a low moan, laying his head back down on the slick cold cement.

"Shhh, hold still boy, help is coming."

A tattered blue collar hung around his long neck. He belonged to someone, someone who would be heartbroken that their beloved dog had suffered and who would feel guilty because they had not been there for him when he needed comfort. He heaved one big breath, in then out, and blood flowed from his mouth over the moist pink skin of his lip, trailing down the gutter with the rainwater. His luminous green eyes were glazed and fixed. I continued to talk to him, even though I was pretty sure he could no longer hear my words.

"It's okay boy, it's okay now. I'm here. I'm so sorry, boy. I'm sorry, I'm so sorry." I sobbed on my knees beside him.

The sound of tires approaching and the flash of headlights startled me to my feet. A car pulled up, the door of the small SUV opened and a tall, slender woman walked towards me.

"Are you alright," she asked? "Is this your dog?"

"No, he's not mine. He was hit by a car and everyone left. They just drove away."

Stepping forward, arms outstretched, the kind stranger wrapped me in a warm hug and I collapsed in her arms. She took a step back, her hands cupping my shoulders, bracing me, and looked me in the face. "Oh honey, that's awful," she said, "He doesn't look like he is going to make it."

I nodded. "I think he stopped breathing a few minutes ago."

"I have a blanket in my truck," she said, "Let's cover him up." I followed closely behind her as she continued to gently talk to me.

"I'm a nurse at Mission Hospital, so I carry blankets and a first aid kit. If he is still alive, he is in shock. We need to cover him up so he doesn't become hypothermic."

I shuddered and nodded in agreement, but did not offer that I had intimate knowledge on the subjects—shock, hypothermia, and death. Somewhere on the walk back to the dog we introduced ourselves, and shared that we both had dogs of our own, speculating how sad the owner would be to hear about the accident. We each took a corner of the blanket and draped it down across the dog's shoulders just beneath his silky black ears, leaving his beautiful boxy head exposed.

He hadn't moved for a very long time when the animal control truck finally came wheeling around the median, tires screeching on the wet pavement like an ambulance arriving at an emergency. The uniformed driver burst from his vehicle towards us, loaded for bear.

"Which one of you did this?" he screamed indignantly, pointing down at the blanket.

My head dropped, my shoulders caved, and I began to cry all over again. Feeling choked by my misplaced guilt, I gulped in a deep breath and felt something start to burn and swell in my chest. I could not contain it. I had finally had enough guilt and blame. I raised my chin and met his gaze. "This is not my fault, I did nothing." I shrieked. "I didn't do it, I DIDN'T DO IT."

The woman who carried blankets in her car sweetly stepped into my defense. "He was hit by a car and everyone drove off. She stayed behind with him."

The officer's demeanor instantly softened; he stuttered out an apology and went to work. The young man bent down, pulling the blanket back slightly as he placed two fingers on the dog's neck, holding them there for a few seconds. Shaking his head in disgust, he acknowledged what I already knew. The officer tenderly pushed the dog's eyelids closed and swept the animal's limp body up, head and tail hanging over his cradled arms, carrying him back to the truck, and deposited him into one of the small holding compartments. I thanked the officer for his help as he jumped back into his truck to leave. I hugged my guardian angel nurse, thanking her for staying with me, and watched her drive down the street until her taillights disappeared into the darkness.

Walking back to my car, I paused under the streetlight, and leaned my head back while the drizzle cooled the hot tears that dripped down my face. I breathed in the fresh moist air, the first real breath I had taken in four years, and began my apology.

"I'm sorry I wasn't there for you, Mom. I did the best that I could do. It is time for me to let this go or I will drown in the sorrow, the grief, and the guilt."

The rain began to pour. I shoved my hand in my pocket, searching for my car keys and glanced down at the pavement where the stray had taken his final breath, the asphalt still stained in red. And I stood there on the damp street staring at that spot until the last drops of blood washed away down the gutter and the stream of water finally ran clear.

Epilogue

In the years after Mom died, I focused on getting my own mental health in order. I began to see a new therapist and became acutely aware of all the people who live with anxiety and depression, post-traumatic stress disorder, panic attacks, and other disorders. I was diagnosed with dysthymia, a mild, but chronic form of depression, post-traumatic stress, and ADHD, which was quite a revelation. I saw in myself what I had begun to see all around me—people suffering in silence because they were too embarrassed to be honest and upfront about their mental health. Sue, who had been such a rock of support for me during my grieving, was one of those people.

★   ★   ★

Even before I answered the buzzing cell phone tucked in the pocket of my pajama bottoms, I knew something was terribly wrong. I had somehow become an expert at "terribly wrong." It was as if I had developed a new sense that could determine whether something was just run-of-the-mill wrong, or really truly, life-alteringly bad, and my gut told me this phone call was bad. My dear friend Sue was in trouble.

She had been struggling for months. The change in her was subtle, at first. Once a vibrant, tall, gorgeous, redhead with a lightning fast, razor-sharp wit, and a vocabulary that would make Webster proud, my friend lost her confidence, then headed face first into a downward spiral of depression. She started to question every decision she made, especially ones about her parenting, ruminating over and over again about whether or not she had done the right thing. Sue was driven to be a great mother, but she began to compare her style and her resolve to others. In her own eyes, she did not measure up because Sue believed that she was too inconsistent and lacked the backbone to stand up to her teenagers. But Sue did not have *bad* kids; in fact, Cassidy and Bennett were amazing, model children who excelled in school and sports. They could be challenging at times, like teenagers can be, but were respectful and engaging the great majority of the time.

It had only been a few months since I had begun to notice the troubles in Sue's marriage and the depression that kicked in as a result, but as the holidays approached, Sue's state of mind became much more obvious to everyone. As she withdrew from friends and social gatherings, they began to ask me, "Is everything okay with Sue?" I would lamely say, "Yes, she is fine," but to close friends I would describe her state as someone trying to climb a greased slide; she could not get her footing and I secretly feared how far she would slip.

As I watched my friend free fall into the abyss of major depression, I felt helpless to slow her decent, and a stifling cloud of dread swooped in over me. I hadn't been able to help my mother, but surely I could help Sue. She had been there for me when I was held prisoner by my own grief, depression, and guilt after my mom's death. Sue was one of the few people who could relate to losing their mother without warning, and her wisdom and friendship helped me understand and pull through my own grief.

I didn't recognize what was wrong with my mother until it was too late, but it was clear to me that Sue was in a deep depression, sinking further every day, and it was brutal to watch. I desperately asked my therapist, Rosemary, how to help, what to ask, where to take Sue, and I did everything she suggested, but nothing I said or did altered Sue's course, her thinking, or her feelings, about herself. She was completely overwhelmed by every aspect of her day.

At the end of January, after weeks of cheerleading, telling her I believed she could handle all that was on her plate, I had to face the fact that she could not. Sue's family realized the gravity of her condition as well, and Sue's brother, Richard, an Orange County sheriff, stepped in to help make the decision to take Sue to the hospital for evaluation and counseling—not a 5150 psychiatric hold, which would hospitalize Sue against her will, but a voluntary admission to the hospital; she wanted to go and she needed to go. Sue could not stand the thought of telling her children such frightening news. She was overwhelmed with embarrassment and felt ashamed by the perception that she was too weak because she could not simply will herself out of her depression and be there for her kids.

Sue tortured herself, asking me repeatedly, "What kind of mother chooses to leave her children?"

"It's only for three days, Susie." I answered, but her look of despair told me she was unconvinced.

So we made a plan: the kids would be spared the exact details of a psychiatric hospitalization and would be told that their mother was going to the hospital for an evaluation because she had been losing weight, was feeling "sad" and unable to sleep. Our friend Gina picked the kids up after school, I handled things at the house, and Richard took his little sister to the hospital.

Later that afternoon, Richard asked me to put together an overnight bag for Sue, so I rummaged through Sue's clothes in the large walk-in closet in her bedroom. It was half empty. A month earlier, her husband had taken his clothes, and Sue found it unbearable to even be in that space. Sue and I were close friends, yet I felt as though I was somehow violating her privacy searching through her lingerie drawer in that highly charged atmosphere. *What do you wear in the psychiatric ward?* I thought, as I hastily tossed sweats, T-shirts and toiletries into a duffle bag. Intuition struck me over the head when I got into my car to drive, and I dialed the hospital for instructions.

"South Coast Medical," the operator cheerily answered.

"Hello," I said, "May I speak to someone in the psychiatry ward, please?"

They transferred me. "Behavioral Health, may I help you?"

"Um, yes," I stumbled, "I have a friend staying there, and I am bringing her some clothing and personal items. Do you have some recommendations or guidelines for what I should bring her?"

As I suspected and quickly discovered, nearly everything I had packed for Sue with the exception of her underwear would not be allowed because it would be deemed unsafe by the hospital staff. They would carefully examine every item before handing it over to a patient, and I was told something like sweat pants was a no-go. I had been politely instructed not to bring anything with a drawstring, laces, or belt because of their potential risk to Sue and others on the floor—running shoes, out; hooded sweatshirt, out; robe, out; drawstring sweats, out.

In addition, I was told no sharp objects (not even a nail clipper) and no drugs or alcohol (which seemed quite obvious). I hung up with the nurse on duty and quickly ran to Target to shop for acceptable, comfortable things for Sue to wear. Months later, I would become disconcerted when I saw Sue in the clothes I had picked for her hospital stay, like when you hear a song that floods you with memories of a bad breakup and are instantly filled with heartache.

The past six years had been a tidal wave of fear and anxiety, and as much as I had grown accustomed to the feeling, I could not shake the weight of melancholy and tight grasp of panic that seized me as I walked through the doors of the Behavioral Health Services unit. My stomach turned as I noted the heavy steel doors and reinforced glass. No one was going in or out of this place without permission. It was not your typical floor at the hospital, bustling with pleasant nurses and kind volunteers with floral deliveries and magazines for the patients, and I could not for the life of me imagine why someone would ask to stay here.

I approached the closed window and stood for a few minutes until I was acknowledged by a somber-looking woman from inside the office. She casually quizzed me about every item in the bag, and when satisfied with my description of the contents, sent a gentleman out to retrieve it from me. The thick door buzzed as it opened and I could see down the long hallway where a patient leaned, legs crossed, intently and nervously talking on a pay phone. *Where is Sue?* I thought, overcome by the desire to rush in, scream her name and rescue her from this awful scary place. *How could being here possibly feel better than being at home?* In that moment, I knew there was something I did not fully understand about what my friend was going through. I expected her to think and reason in the same way as me but something was standing in her way . . . and I desperately wanted to move it for her.

I went home, feeling totally powerless. All I could do for the next few days was hope and pray.

★   ★   ★

On Friday, four days later, Sue was released from the hospital in spite of the fact that she felt no better than when she had checked in, but Sue was determined to get home to her kids. We ate lunch at a local restaurant and I stayed with her at her house that afternoon because she was still dreadfully depressed. The last thing

I told Sue when I hugged her goodbye was, "I love you, and if you get in your car, drive down to my house." I didn't want her to be alone, but she assured me she was okay.

Saturday morning, I texted Sue at 9:20 a.m., just to let her know I was thinking about her. By 10:00 a.m. I had not heard back from her—and that was when I began to get the sure sense that something wasn't right. An hour passed. My daughter, Katy, and I were mid-conversation when I pulled the vibrating BlackBerry up closer to my face to get a good look at the screen. I gasped, and pushed the button.

"Hello, " I said, barely getting the two words out before Sue's husband hit me with a short barrage of questions.

"Where is she?" he asked impatiently, in a panicked and indignant tone. I assumed he was talking about Sue.

"I don't know. I haven't spoken with her yet this morning."

"Oh, so *you* didn't call Cassidy?" he asked.

"No," I said, and was about to explain that I had not called their teenage daughter, when the line went dead.

I frantically dialed Gina's number. A second later and with not so much as a "Hello," Gina began pouring out the conversation she had just had with Cassidy. "Sue's in the emergency room at Mission Hospital. Her brother is there, and she is talking. She was in a car accident."

Worn out from the months of worry and anxiety about what I knew was happening to my friend and was powerless to stop, I stood frozen with fear. "Oh my God, is she going to be okay?" I asked feebly.

"I don't . . . know," Gina said.

Pulling on my jeans with one hand, my throat began to close and the tears poured out. Gina said she would pick up Cassidy and then me on her way to the hospital.

Katy stood with me as I struggled into my clothes and her pained expression implored me to explain what was happening. I hung up and told her the little I knew from my brief conversation.

"Sue has been in a car accident. Gina and Cassidy are picking me up in a few minutes so we can take Cassidy to see her mom in the emergency room."

"Was it really an accident, Mom?" Katy asked, about to cry herself. I had been honest with Katy about how Sue was feeling and why she needed her friends more than ever.

"I don't know, Sweetie." I said, but I *did* know, in my heart.

Gina took Cassidy up to Sue's room a few minutes ahead of me. When I finally stepped inside the elevator, I felt as if my body had been injected with Novocain; I actually felt nothing. I pushed the button and tried to imagine what I would say when I got to Sue's hospital room. Numb with fear and trepidation about what I was about to walk into, I ran the scenes of the last few months through my head, watching each floor number illuminate on the impossibly slow ride up and realized I had nothing to say. I was speechless . . . but angry. *At whom?* I thought. The bing of the elevator startled me to my core. I forced myself to step out between the open doors and down the long hallway, fighting my conflicting desires to flee from the scene and rush down the hall to see Sue.

I pushed the door open to find Cassidy keenly focused on Sue's bruised face. Sue's nose was clearly broken and her lip was as swollen as I have ever seen a lip—fat and purple, like a ripe plum. Staring down at the hospital blanket draped over one leg, Sue glanced up at me for a split second and quickly looked away, but I caught the flash of guilt and shame in her eyes. Sue turned her focus back to the thermal hospital blanket that she clung to while the doctors and nurses moved about the room around her. I saw something else in her once vibrant eyes: anger, despair, and pain—not pain from the discomfort of her injuries, but the kind of pain that comes from being so deeply ashamed and consumed with self-loathing that you want to crawl out of your skin and disappear.

I was unbelievably thankful Sue was alive, but could not linger in my joy for long. There was no place for it in Sue's small hospital room, which was shrouded in overwhelming sadness and confusion. Sue was lucky to be alive. She had suffered extensive injuries, but I knew as she lay there, she felt anything but lucky.

I stepped away down the hall to be alone and placed a call to my therapist, Rosemary, and asked her to phone me back immediately. Rosemary knew Sue because they had spoken on a few occasions and I had been keeping her abreast of Sue's progress. The minute I answered my phone and heard her voice, I began to sob.

"Lauri, are you okay?" she asked.

"No, it's Sue. She is in the hospital and she tried to take her own life today," I blurted out through my tears.

"Oh, Lauri, I am so very sorry."

"Please, you have to tell me that Sue can recover from this, please," I begged through my tears. "I cannot lose someone else like this, I can't do it. Tell me you have treated patients that have done this and are living happy full lives now."

"Yes, Sue has experienced a major depressive episode, but I have treated many, many patients who have been where she is today. It's not going to be easy, but it is entirely possible for Sue to recover."

Over the next few days, Sue underwent major surgery, daily changes to her anti-depressant medications, and had to endure a barrage of uncomfortable questions and conversations with doctors, friends, and family about what had happened. She was beyond humiliated. Everywhere I turned, there was conversation about Sue. "How could Sue have been so selfish or so weak?

Other people are having marital problems and they're just fine. How could Sue do this to her kids, to her family, and to her friends?" I began to feel sick from the poisonous gossip and speculation that was being cavalierly spread around town about my friend.

Sue lay in a hospital bed, helpless to defend herself, all the while she ruminated about what people were saying, and rightly so. Everyone had an opinion about what Sue needed to do, what she "should" do, how she should be treated. How could Sue possibly recover in the face of such judgment and self-righteousness? *No wonder people do not seek treatment or talk openly about their struggles or triumphs with mental illness*, I thought. There is simply too much judgment and stigma, and too little compassion and empathy associated with this illness. Why is mental illness treated differently than any other illness? Because it can be scary and people do not understand it. I did not understand it myself.

After Sue's accident, I spoke with Rosemary often because I had to. I needed to understand mental illness, both Sue's and my mother's. They had different diagnoses; a mood disorder versus a personality disorder. But their brain disorders had convinced them both that death was the only option left to them. It wasn't a lack of effort or because of weakness, or because they are selfish. And it certainly wasn't because of something I had done or had not done. It wasn't about me. It was about the illness.

I visited Sue regularly in the hospital, but not every day. I couldn't do it. The emotional toll was just too heavy, a harsh reminder of the feelings I hadn't properly dealt with after my mom's death. Initially I had been angry at Sue, and as much as I didn't want to think about it, I was still angry at my mom. After the case was closed, I rushed to put my feelings away because I had spent four hard years investigating and grieving a murder. I felt relieved that the hunt for the truth was finally over. And I needed to move forward.

But I hadn't let go of my resentment towards my mom for the pain that her suicide had caused our family. I hadn't allowed myself to contemplate her suicide. It was too painful and I'd had enough pain.

Standing over Susie as she lay in the hospital bed, broken in every way possible, suffering in the deepest pain and sadness I have ever personally witnessed, and battling relentless shame and guilt, reminded me of a promise I had made to myself when I heard that Mom had been murdered: I vowed that I would make something good happen from Mom's death—*big* good.

Investigating my mother's death was an empowering journey for me. In the process I learned to speak up for myself and my mom, asking questions and demanding answers, and found a voice inside of me that had been silent for too long. As I stood in Sue's hospital room, it was clear as ever to me what my big good would be: I would use my voice to help free my friend of the shame and guilt she carried simply because she was sick. No one should feel ashamed of having an illness, just because it cannot be seen on an x-ray. Although Sue's future was still uncertain, and her family, friends, and I were unsure of exactly how to help, I was certain I wanted to be there for Sue on her journey back, just as she has been there for me.

Late one afternoon about a week after the car crash, I was sitting alone in an armchair tucked in the corner of Sue's stark room, watching her sleep. She had arrived battered in the emergency room, but her lip was finally beginning to settle down, and she had started physical therapy to learn to use a wheel chair. Sue began to stir uncomfortably in the steel framed hospital bed, and opened her eyes. I gently grabbed the rail, pulling on the bar to steady myself and stood up close to the bed near her shoulder.

"Hi," I said, softly, smiling down at her.

"Hi, Laur," she said, barely a whisper, blinking her eyes closed for a moment and spoke again when she opened them.

"Laur, I am so sorry I put you through all this," Sue said, pausing, drawing in a shallow breath, which she slowly breathed out before she continued, "after everything you have been through with your mom."

Her words caught me off guard and lay like stone, heavy on my chest. My heart ached as if my mother had just spoken an apology to me herself—it ached because of how much I'd needed to hear the apology and because of how much the apology had cost. As I looked into Sue's misty eyes, which were draped in sadness, regret, and remorse, my own eyes filled to the brim. "Thank you, Susie," I said, my tears dripping down over the tip of my nose onto the sheets as I reached over to lay my hand on top of hers. "I accept your apology . . . I forgive you."

But I knew in my heart there was nothing to forgive. Sue hadn't done anything to me, or to her friends or to her family. The truth was this had happened to *her.* Just like it had happened to my mom.

Sue was exhausted from her physical therapy, from the shame that she struggled with every minute of every day, and from the worry about what she was going to face when she was released from the hospital.

"Close your eyes, Susie, everything is going to be okay," I said, squeezing her hand, "I'm not going anywhere."

"I love you, Laur," she whispered, closing her eyes.

"I love you, too," I said.

Life gives us gifts wrapped in the strangest paper—and mine came wrapped in tragedy. The life changing events of Sue's major depressive episode and attempted suicide allowed me to look through the lens of her experience to finally learn about and understand with greater compassion why my mom had taken that last desperate step on a desolate stretch of Baja coastline. There was no crime. It wasn't her fault, and finally, with enormous relief, I realized that it wasn't mine either.

About the Author

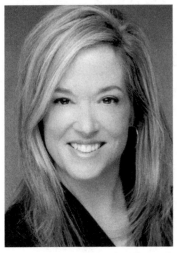

Steven Khan Photography

Lauri Taylor spent nearly four years investigating her mother's murder in both the United States and Mexico, but before that she was a marketing and branding expert who worked with professional athletes and premium lifestyle brands. She worked with NBA professionals developing their unique brand identities through endorsement opportunities, speaking engagements, public appearances and philanthropic associations. Her work in the field has also included event marketing and implementation, in which she partnered with corporate clients at major sporting events to increase brand awareness and consumer loyalty through advertising, media coverage and social opportunities for customers and employees.

Lauri has lived with anxiety, depression, and post-traumatic stress and has become an advocate for shameless communication about mental health and the stigma of mental illness. *The Accidental Truth* is her first book.

Lauri is a graduate of SMU's Cox School of Business, holding a Bachelor of Business Administration degree, with a major in marketing and a minor in Spanish. She lives in Orange County, California and is the mother of two grown children. She is a member of the SMU Alumni Association, the Cox School of Business Alumni Association, and the National Charity League.